LIVE,

LAUGH, and

LOVE with

DEMENTIA

D1056691

by Luann R. Sackrider

ISBN: 1494459078

This book is dedicated to caregivers everywhere.

May you find **laughter** as you endure one of life's deepest, darkest pits.

May you learn, as Betsie & Corrie Ten Boom did in Ravensbruck death camp,

"There is no pit so deep that God's love is not deeper still."

And in the end, may you hear Him whisper in your ear,

"Well done, good and faithful servant." Matthew 25:23

ACKNOWLEDGEMENTS

After being in the classroom for over 25 years and our family's subsequent move to Colorado in 2009, I had a weird, nagging sense that I needed to fulfill some "greater purpose" in my life. I thought that was in the classroom, but, as I write this book, I realize this book is what the nagging sense was all about. And it is my hope that sharing our family's experiences with dementia will help others.

I wish to thank my family for their willingness to open our home to my mother in the first place. Pete, Jessica, and I were a team and constant support to one another. I truly thank God for them.

I wish to thank my mother and father for their constant love, support, and sense of security which they provided me over 50 some years. I wouldn't be the person I am today without them. My mother would always tell me as a child, I was going to "drive her demented," which I never quite understood. In the end, she did become demented, and it was my honor to be there to love and care for her.

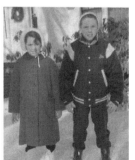

Christmas, 1963

I would also like to acknowledge my students who kept me grounded, focused, and gave me great joy during this difficult journey during the two years Mom lived with us in Hawaii. They also helped me with Mom on a few occasions when I had to bring her to school. I can still envision those tender moments as my 10-year-old students took Mom by the hand and helped her get places within the building---priceless. They truly demonstrated one of our school philosophies, "Whenever you can, help." Also, to the administrators at my private school who always supported me in "taking care of family first" as emergencies arose, thank you.

I wish to thank the adult center in Hawaii which gave Mom a safe, loving place to be each day. They planned activities and kept daily routines which continued to stimulate her mind, and the routines made her comfortable.

I would like to thank Dr. Mark for his kindness and professionalism while caring for Mom. He still is passionate about internal medicine and helping his patients. His guidance and wisdom continues to this day.

Thanks to Pam and Gretchen who gave thoughtful advice regarding this book and also, Alphagraphics of Aurora, Colorado who helped me in countless ways. Maureen, a high school friend, created the sassy ladybug. And Ron for his wise counsel.

I don't believe in coincidence, which is what some would say when I ran into Diana, our family friend and colleague, at a recent college reunion. As we caught up with one another, she shared that she had recently lost her dad to Alzheimer's disease. Thank you for your time and help in seeing this book to fruition. Your guidance and expertise in helping edit this book honors your personal experience with this disease, as well as the hope of finding a cure.

Many other people who came alongside of us, such as friends who would take Mom to play cards, to a church event, to a movie, for a ride on a golf cart, or stop by just to say, "Hello". There were those who agreed to be on Mom's emergency contact list at the adult day care center. But the two people who were always there when we needed them most were Jim and Diane who were our rock! Not to mention, the angels that surrounded us...

Contents

Preface

So who was this woman I affectionately called "Mom" before this terrible disease robbed her of her personhood?

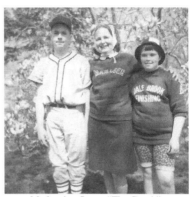

My brother Steve, "The Coach", Mom and me

Mom's nickname was "Junebug," which also led to a love of anything with a ladybug design. In high school she was the drum majorette and valedictorian of her class. In adulthood Mom was always an active community member. She was a member of the Jaycees and volunteered in the PTA and Girl Scouts and coached my softball team. She worked periodically during my childhood at several insurance companies. In retirement her hobbies included traveling, golfing, crossword puzzles, playing bridge, and shopping. In fact, she occasionally indulged in "depression shopping." I was with her on one such occasion when she traded up one diamond ring for another, "Just because!" On another shopping trip she happened to be in a Macy's store in the Washington, D.C. area on 9/11. When Macy's announced why they would be closing the store at noon, she went on a shopping spree thinking that the world might well end. Or perhaps she was pre-depression shopping!

Mom was a natural teacher and responsible for my success in school. She and my dad practiced the best of "tough love" before it was popular! Mom monitored my schoolwork closely and never let me slack off.

She was known for her engaging personality, love of life,

11

and sense of humor. Her philosophy of life was to thank God everyday when you wake up and to be thankful for friends, family, and your health. She was a devoted wife, mother, and grandmother.

After Mom had lived with us in Hawaii for two of our five years there, we prepared to move to Colorado and make the change then, under the advice of our family doctor, to move her to an assisted living facility. The headmaster at the school where I taught knew Mom briefly but only knew her with dementia. He had these parting words, "Best wishes to your mom as well. She has always been quick to smile when we have chatted, and, even as she ages, she retains a special charm evident to those of us who only knew her casually."

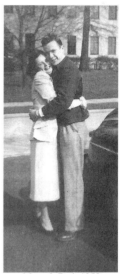

Mom & Dad, 1950

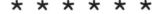

The setting for this story takes place mainly between the years 2003-2010. For many years my mom and our family resided within a few miles from one another in Annapolis, Maryland. In 2004 our family moved to Kapolei, Hawaii, but we traveled to Annapolis regularly to see Mom. After she suffered a stroke in 2007, Mom came to live with us in Hawaii. In 2009 we moved to Aurora, Colorado; us, to a new home, and Mom, to an "assisted living" home for people with dementia.

The medical information in this book is not intended as medical advice. Consult your health care provider.

The legal information in this book is not intended as legal advice. Consult your family or estate lawyer and the laws that apply in the state where you reside.

And finally, this book was written to provide laughter to caregivers, not to poke fun at my mom or this horrible disease. Remember, many of these stories were NOT funny to us at the time!

No less than 20% of the net proceeds of this book will be donated to Alzheimer's research in hopes of a cure before we are victims of this horrible, personality-altering disease. Current research suggests that one out of two baby boomers who live to age 85 will be victims of this disease.

So, above all, may you

LIVE, LAUGH, and LOVE with Dementia.

"Every experience God gives us,

every person He puts in our lives,

is the perfect preparation for

a future only He can see."

Corrie Ten Boom

Chapter 1
OUR LIVES FOREVER CHANGED

This is our story, one of many stories with no two a
It is the story of how our lives were changed forev
that day on September 8 when my mother came for
a "three month visit" to get back on her feet after
suffering a stroke on August 5, 2007. The stroke
occurred on the right side of her brain, which affec
all of the left side of her body. She had to relearn h
to walk, talk, and use her arm again. Remarkably, wit
time, there were no residual effects from the strok
physically, except for the dementia.

My husband Pete, daughter Jessica, and I just happe
to be on vacation in July 2007 visiting my mom in
Annapolis, Maryland, our hometown as well. We were
living in Hawaii on a five year work assignment from
2004-'09 and were "home" for a two week vacation,
which turned into six weeks away due to two trips to t
hospital with Mom.

First, Mom was hospitalized in July 2007 for a flesh tea
of her leg so deep we were told that there was a fifty
percent chance of losing her leg. This was due to her
complex health history of diabetes, high blood pressure,
peripheral artery disease (PAD), stroke, and ulcerated
colitis. Three days after leaving the hospital, she
suffered the stroke. Thankfully, we were visiting her
when the stroke occurred and called 911.* We were able
to get her the risky clot busting drug, tissue plasminogen
activator (tPA)** which helped her totally recover
physically from the stroke. She stayed another week in
the hospital and then at a rehabilitation facility for three
weeks of physical therapy. What we were not prepared
for was that the stroke increased her mild memory
issues. It had its upside though. She suddenly didn't

em to have a care in the world and had a more "go with
e flow" attitude!

s a teacher, I had the summer off; our daughter
essica had summer break from the University of
awaii; and my husband Pete utilized the Family and
edical Leave Act*** due to the fact that our two
eek vacation turned into a six week stint. Mom was so
touch and go" that Pete was afraid to go back to Hawaii
nly to have to return for a funeral. After she went to
he rehabilitation facility, we returned to Hawaii. Pete
greed to go and get her from the rehabilitation facility
n Maryland to bring her to Hawaii, as I had just begun
a new school year. For three months we agreed to care
or Mom in our two bedroom, 850 sq. ft. condo! Jessica
willingly gave up her bedroom for this undertaking.
Surely, we could do anything for three months.

So this is the story of how three months turned into
over three years. Too many books tell you all the horrible
things about dementia. I call them "Debbie Downer"
books. I hope this book gives those who are caring for
a loved one with dementia ideas as to how to LIVE your
life, keeping things as normal as possible, while caring for
a loved one with memory loss. The LOVE part of the title
in this book refers to what you are already doing – family
takes care of family. It's that simple- unconditional love-
period. And, LAUGH… find the humor. It is certainly not
my intention to offend anyone by writing about some of
our experiences or to laugh at this horrible disease. I do,
however, hope that you may see the humorous situations
as you give care through some very dark times.

As the dementia progressed, our family took great
pride in telling my mother tall tales, which were also a
barometer of how her brain was on any given day. One
of our favorite tall tales was when we would tell her that

Pete's mom was coming down for "the surgery." She would ask, "What surgery?" We would then explain that she and Pete's mom were donating their extra breast tissue to Jess and me! They were getting reductions; we were getting enlargements! If she

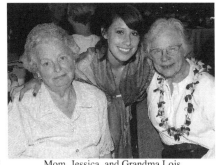

Mom, Jessica, and Grandma Lois

responded, "You're full of sh--!" to this tale, then that was a good brain day. If she went along with this crazy story, then that was a not-so-good brain day. And there were other things she did to make us laugh as well.

Of course, the last three years were not a picnic. There were really stressful moments, but we were fortunate that Mom was generally happy and content. She worked hard to act as though she was "with it." In hindsight, the past three years were the most difficult yet rewarding three years of our lives. But after all Mom had sacrificed for me over the years, it was the least I could do for her. Pete, Jessica, and I grew closer as a family, closer to God, and relied more upon one another. So, would I (we) do it all again? Yes, family takes care of family. PERIOD.

 HELPFUL HINTS

* When paramedics arrived, I dutifully pulled out my new Health Insurance Portability and Accountability Act (HIPAA) document stating she was a Do Not Resuscitate (DNR) and I was her representative. They responded that the HIPAA document only applied once she was at the hospital. If she went into cardiac arrest on her way to the hospital, they would have to revive her. The document I needed and didn't have was an original copy

of Emergency Medical Services (EMS) and Do Not Resuscitate (DNR) Medical Care Order provided by the state. It states your wishes specifically, such as DNR, for emergency personnel. You can get this free of charge at your doctor's office. The three states we lived in with Mom all had them: Maryland, Hawaii, and Colorado. The document should be posted on the refrigerator, and emergency personnel are trained to look there for it.

**tPA- Tissue Plasminogen Activator must be administered within a few hours after documenting a stroke or heart attack has occurred. It breaks up the clot which caused the event. The use of tPA can be fatal.

***Family and Medical Leave Act of 1993 (signed by President Clinton) provides up to 12 weeks of unpaid, job-protected leave per year while caring for a family member and other personal or family related medical situations.

Hindsight really is 20/20. Looking back, there were many signs along the way that Mom was in the beginning stage of dementia.

In July 2010 we finally got around to cleaning out her home in preparation to sell it. We were surprised to find literature that she had received from the Alzheimer's Foundation dated 1992. I don't know if she was concerned about herself or, more likely, my dad. He, however, did not have dementia, just "selective memory."

Mom had moved to live near us in Annapolis, MD, in 1998 because she wanted to live near family... and die near family. She even bought a new condo, thinking that the new appliances would last 12 years or until the end of her life. And it was exactly that long - 12 years.

As I look back, I think 2003 was the year things started. I remember her calling me from her home one day. We lived, as my husband would say, 5.2 miles apart. Mom was crying because she had not been able to find her car in a parking lot. I asked where she was and she replied, "Home." I asked her how she got there, and she said some "nice man" helped her find her car. (She was always charming some nice man.)

Another thing we found while cleaning out her home in July 2010 were two driver's licenses neatly tucked away in a wallet in a dresser drawer. They had been "lost", and one was issued in April of '03 and the other in June of '03! The current license she had been using was issued in November of '06. I am not sure if there were others. Perhaps she misplaced a license while showing it to the "nice man", in, I believe, '04, who pulled her over for speeding. He was a nice man – he only gave her a warning ticket although she was driving nearly 20 mph over the limit!

Another sign was when she switched investment firms out of the blue. When she came to live with us, I knew I should be added onto that account, in case of an emergency, and discovered that mom had not even listed my brother or me as beneficiaries. No beneficiaries were listed at all! That is a detail that would not have been overlooked in the past. Mom also stopped balancing her checkbook, which is particularly interesting because she was an excellent mathematician. Actually, my mother was one of the smartest people I have ever known.

Then there was the time we went to the local grocery store to pick up a few things on her grocery list. She was always highly organized. As we checked out, she pulled out her credit card. Then she said excitedly, "Watch this!" She entered the appropriate codes and added the cash back option. The clerk handed her the receipt with $20, and as we walked away, she whispered, "Not only do they give you your groceries, they pay you to shop here!" I knew she normally kept a tight budget with her monthly income, but she was no longer keeping track of her credit cards. Mom had her main bills on auto pay so she had to stay within her budget, not wanting to cash in her investments. I think it was around 2006 when this lack of budgeting and "free grocery trips" came to a head. We were visiting her for Christmas and noticed that she had several overdrawn notices from the bank! This had never happened before, and it wasn't that she didn't have money but rather not enough in the account from which the bills were automatically being paid.

Speaking of bills, my mother had the "I've fallen and can't get up" type alert program offered through our local electric company. She wore a simple bracelet while home so if she fell, she could speak into a voice box and help would come. One day she was having trouble understanding the billing so she phoned the company. After calling several times and being put on an automated system, she grew frustrated. Then it occurred to her that if she pushed the button on the bracelet, a person would talk to her and perhaps answer her billing questions...and so she did! Well, did that backfire! It is just like calling 911, and you can't undo it! An ambulance was dispatched, even though she tried to tell the person speaking from the voice box that it was not an emergency just a billing question! When my husband and I found out about this event we were furious! We explained that not only were thousands of tax dollars wasted but someone else could have died by not receiving aid. I helped her find out where the ambulance was dispatched from, took her in person to apologize, and had her bring food to the fire station as well. Perhaps this was the beginning of when things began to come "full circle", and I started to parent my parent.

Another clue was that during one of the times we were visiting Mom in Annapolis after we had moved to Hawaii in 2004, we noticed she was not as organized or bothered by our usual mess. Since the condo was small, we would stay in the small second bedroom, and our suitcases would sit in the dining room. She would usually nag us to keep things exceptionally tidy, but she didn't that trip. If you knew my mom, you would know how significant this was. Her home could pass any white glove test for cleanliness; she was organized throughout the house and wrote everything down. I also noticed that the linen closet was not tidy as usual.

She seemed to no longer be making the usual shopping lists as she had failed to purchase groceries for our arrival but had an abundance of snacks for when she would host bridge in her home. In fact, she seemed to have triple the amount of mints, nuts, crackers, and cookies for bridge. And when we arrived during that same visit, we could smell a strange smell in her hallway outside her condo. My mother had the absolute best sense of smell of anyone I knew. She always said she could, "Smell cow turd a mile away." And, indeed, I think she could. When we went into her condo, the smell grew stronger. She opened the refrigerator, and we almost got sick. She said, "I think there is a dead cat in there", but she didn't have a cat. Upon inspection, we found ground beef that had gone so horribly bad that it had maggots!

My mother took approximately 13 prescriptions, no lie. She knew what every pill was for and when to take it. She took meds for diabetes, blood pressure, heart, and ulcerative colitis, among others. When hospitalized, she would argue that the hospital schedule of giving meds at 10:00 am and 10:00 pm was not how her meds should be taken, and she was right. The nurses got so tired of hearing her complain that they would allow her to bring in her pills, which were in am and pm organizers, and take them herself!

But certainly by 2006 she was no longer taking her pills as prescribed. She could no longer organize them in weekly pill containers or name them all. She would leave all the pill bottles on the counter and take them sporadically, which was fast becoming a problem. My mother, being a stroke risk, was on the drug Coumadim also known as Warfarin, which is used to prevent blood clots or to keep clots from growing larger. She convinced her doctor that she could just use Plavix (to keep plaque from forming) to prevent stroke, which was totally misguided. This was not a realistic choice for her with her existing health issues. Both medicines performed different, needed functions, and a couple of months after taking herself off Coumadin, she suffered a severe stroke. Besides not setting up her pill container, I also noticed she wasn't drinking coffee but rather tea. I later realized the she had forgotten how to make coffee.

Another thing I noticed during my 2007 visit, while I was on spring break from my school in Hawaii, was that Mom eagerly agreed to attend a fundraiser for the school

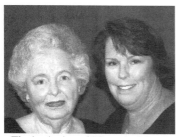

The beginning of "Groucho Marx" eyebrows after I toned them down.

where I had previously worked. This was really out of character as she didn't like late nights and kept a pretty busy schedule for herself. We had fun getting, as Mom would say, all "gussied up" while picking out out similar black cocktail dresses to wear. Next, we chose her jewelry, and finally just the right shoes. She put on her makeup and what a surprise that was! The eyebrows were a bit "Groucho Marxish" and needed to be toned down! We did, however, really enjoy the evening together with her new "go with the flow" attitude.

Yes, there were signs, but since we were living far away in Hawaii during the early stages of her disease, they were difficult to detect. She was still active in two bridge clubs, reading, socializing, playing golf, doing crossword puzzles, and driving.

In the early stages the signs are far more subtle and can be confused with the natural signs of aging and forgetfulness. However, the sooner the diagnosis, the sooner you may be able to start dementia meds which can help your loved one. I am grateful for my mother's very gradual decline, which I believe was due in part to the medicines Aricept and Namenda.

HELPFUL HINTS

Any change in usual pattern can be significant.

Ask your loved one's closest friends if they have noticed any changes in behavior. In particular, are social dates being kept?

Ask questions such as the date, the President, anniversary date, etc. Try to sandwich them in questions that make them appear discreet.

Can they repeat their address and phone number?

Are they keeping doctor, hair, and social appointments?

If you live nearby, look to see if there is a change in how they keep house.

If they take regular meds, check to see if they are being taken.

If you are a joint owner on banking accounts, check on them.

How's their driving? Jessica took the last death-defying drive with my mother. Not only did she cut corners and drive up on curbs, she parked in the loading zone at the grocery store. Jess explained that she could not park there, but my mom insisted that they would soon be loading groceries, so it was "OK." Somehow Jess did convince her to use a parking spot.

A friend who was a nurse once told me about a simple test for dementia which I never tried. She said to put the person in a corner and tell them to find their way out.

Chapter 3
HOSPITAL TRIPS

Unfortunately, if your loved one is elderly, any trip to a hospital, whether for an emergency or elective surgery, is not good. It is the beginning of the end, at least for my Mom.

Anesthesia, which is linked to a temporary Postoperative Cognitive Dysfunction (POCD)*, is now believed to cause a more permanent status in the elderly and those who have dementia. In other words, any time your loved one undergoes surgery with anesthesia, you must weigh the risks of furthering the dementia versus the type of surgery necessary. I wish we had known this.

Mom started having a lot of health issues in 2006. I called Mom on Thanksgiving Day, and she sounded unusually down. In fact, Mom told me she was tired of urinary tract infections and getting old in general. She told me that she told God that she was "ready to die." There was clearly something wrong for a person who loved life. Living approximately 5,000 miles away wasn't helping me figure it out either! Well, it turned out that the urinary tract infection (UTI) had gone septic, infecting the blood stream. A few days after I had spoken with her, she was found on the floor of her condo where she had been unconscious for two days. Friends finally came to check on her after she missed a bridge date, thank God. My brother Steve flew to Annapolis to care for her, and when the IV antibiotics started to work, I asked her about telling God that she wanted to die. She replied, "Oh, I cancelled that prayer!" Thankfully, she recovered from that hospital trip because after the sepsis and being unconscious for two days, the doctors were concerned about her muscle tissue making a full recovery, but that stubborn woman surely did!

In December of 2006, Mom called 911 because she just wasn't "feeling well." When the ambulance came and got her, they were then sent to another hospital because the hospital with all her records was "too full." (I detail this in Chapter 11.) Basically, Mom went into diabetic shock due to waiting in an ER that had no medical records on her. The doctor somehow found my number and called me in Hawaii, and as Mom's HIPAA representative I pleaded with him to get her records from her regular hospital. I got the first flight out the next morning and arrived at the Baltimore area hospital the next day, joined by our son Peter who was living in Massachusetts. Mom was on life support, which would never have happened if they had known her health history. Thankfully, Mom's pastor from her church had been present in Mom's hospital room when I asked the doctor by phone to get her medical records. Thirty hours later, they still had no records, and I was furious. I told them I wanted Mom transferred to her local hospital immediately. Then came a series of stalling answers over a few hours by several doctors. I finally told them that since they never got her medical records and I had a witness to my request, they better get her moved or take the consequences of a malpractice suit. Funny, somehow we were in an ambulance and transferred within the hour.

I wish that was the happy ending to that story, but although Mom got well quickly, our son Peter and I witnessed two aides in another hospital move Mom in her bed which fractured a vertebrae! I promptly spoke with the patient advocate who helped us schedule kyphoplasty surgery, which is a way to treat minor fractures with bone cement. Unfortunately, that couldn't be performed until after the Christmas holidays, but the doctor cleared Mom to travel to Massachusetts so we could spend Christmas with Peter and his new wife Jen.

I wish I could tell you that the kyphoplasty went smoothly, but there were complications. All was going well until some of the glue escaped, which can be deadly, so the procedure was not completed. That night, being playful, we took advantage of Mom coming out of anesthesia and on pain meds. She kept complaining about the compression therapy being used on her legs that would fill up like a blood pressure cuff to keep the circulation going. She kept saying, "Make it stop!" I think this was the original tall tale: we just couldn't help it.

After Mom being so close to death's doorstep during the last two months, we were exhausted. I told her a leprechaun was massaging her legs. Furthermore, I told her that he needed the money to feed his family in Ireland, and we just couldn't ask him to stop. Shortly after she stopped complaining, perhaps believing the story, a dwarf (person of short stature) came in to deliver her dinner. Pete, Jess, and I looked at each other in disbelief as though the joke was on us! Although the procedure was not a complete success, it was a huge relief from pain, and she walked out of the hospital the next day. Unbeknownst to us, more anesthesia and quite possibly further damage to her brain lay ahead.

Mom had multiple vascular procedures performed on her legs, hoping to save them from amputation due to the poor circulation and chronic pain from peripheral artery disease. The first surgery that my brother and I remember for which she went under anesthesia and never fully recovered mentally was in 2007. She had a femoral bypass of the left leg with a cryogenic vein from a forty year old donor. From that day on, Mom liked to brag about having younger "parts" than us!

This is also when a hospitalist told me my mother had

moderate dementia, and I assured her it was the effects of the anesthesia. Mom had been "faking it" in terms of her memory. That doctor changed her diagnosis to mild dementia after some of the anesthesia wore off. We still disagreed with that at the time. However, once you have dealt with the disease personally, you see the early signs in someone else much sooner.

A good doctor is worth his/her weight in gold. Find a doctor, preferably a geriatrician, who will listen to you and your loved one. We met my mother's internist and were never impressed. She once took all her 13 prescriptions in a bag to the doctor to ask if she should be

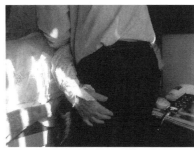
Mom taking advantage of Pete's help.... grabbing his butt!

taking them all. According to Mom, he looked in the bag and said, "They all have your name on them, so I guess so!" They were prescribed by three different doctors, and God only knows what each doctor knew she was taking. Take the medications to your local pharmacy and ask a pharmacist about possible drug interactions. My local pharmacists were a Godsend to me!

 HELPFUL HINTS

*POCD-Postoperative Cognitive Dysfunction-a temporary cognitive decline (brain fog) due to the effects of anesthesia which may be a more permanent cognitive loss in the elderly or those with dementia.

It is important to discuss any recommended surgery with your loved one's doctor and weigh the risks of anesthesia and possibly making their dementia worse as a direct

31

result of anesthesia.

As a caregiver, I suggest you carry a current medicine and health history list with you. Keep a copy for anyone who may substitute for you at times.

Take a list of medicines to your pharmacy and ask the pharmacist to look for drug interactions. This is particularly important if your loved one has more than one doctor.

Chapter 4
PREPARATIONS FOR MOM'S ARRIVAL

We invited Mom to Hawaii in September 2007 for a few months until she regained her strength from the stroke and the severe flesh tear to her leg. She planned to return to Annapolis after the holidays. That being said, we still needed a doctor for the three months. A couple of doctors I asked to take her as a patient would not take her due to her complicated health history, especially short term. But Dr. Mark, our family internist, agreed to help even though his practice was closed to new patients.

So, now that we had a doctor, we still had to administer insulin and wound care to her leg, which her local hospital had taught us how to do. It is particularly difficult for diabetics to heal wounds. The hospital saved Mom's leg and her life, for that matter, with their particular type of silver patch wound care regimen. If Mom's leg had been amputated, she would rather have died and told me this on several occasions. I called around to local medical facilities in Hawaii to see about continuing the wound care. None of the places I called seemed familiar with the products that we were using which were working well. We had been told that there was a 50% chance she would lose her leg from the deep flesh tear. We chose to order the products by mail and continue doing the wound care ourselves. The saline rinse and silver patches saved her leg, and it was completely healed after nine months. They are amazing products, especially for diabetic patients.

The next concern was that stroke patients are likely to experience a stroke again, so we did not feel comfortable leaving her home alone all day. So, we could have paid to have someone come and check in on her, but knowing how social she was, we looked into a nearby adult center which had activities. Remember, we had yet to realize the damage the stroke had done to the brain.

Next, I visited the adult center and wasn't sure it would be ideal, but we didn't have a lot of time to get things set up or consider options for that matter. As an elementary education teacher with special education, I assessed that Mom would certainly be a higher functioning adult there. It was a lengthy process: applying for the adult center, getting medical documents completed in Annapolis, getting a physical and a TB shot. Next, the center needed to interview Mom before starting on Monday, September 10. Thankfully, Nora was willing to meet her on Sunday so we could all get to work on time Monday.

I somewhat regret that we lived with a temporary mindset that Mom would be with us only three months because it held us up from making some timely decisions. After the three months we knew one thing; Mom could not return to her home and live on her own, although she asked us to go back on a regular basis. My brother and I talked about letting her return to Annapolis with help coming in on a regular basis. Pete and I agonized over this but knew her compromised health kept her from realizing her dream of returning home. Any unsupervised time could have put her and others in danger.

Once we came to that conclusion, I should have gotten the Power of Attorney document drawn up. We waited until she was with us for over a year. Had we not waited, we may have been able to sell her condo, which was in a highly sought after retirement community, at the height of the housing market. It was hard getting things done long distance, and we did the best we could, one day at a time.

Next, we had to decide where to put her in our two bedroom condo. Jess generously offered her bedroom, and she agreed to sleep on the couch when she came home from the University of Hawaii on weekends; after all, it was just three months! We realized Mom was used to a firmer bed so we bought a piece of wood to put under the mattress of Jess's couch style daybed. Then we reorganized our small closets, putting things under our bed and in boxes so Mom would have room in Jess's closet. That poor girl pretty much lived out of her boxes which were in the garage during the summers and continued sleeping on the couch for over two years.

Thankfully, our condo was small and had quite a bit of furniture in it already so there weren't a lot of fall risks. If Mom fell she would either fall into a wall or a piece of furniture. So, there was no rearranging to be done. The condo seemed relatively safe, all except the tub style shower. Jess and I helped her get in and out of the shower the first night, and she nearly pulled the two us to the ground. So, the shower situation became Pete's "cross to bear," so to speak!

I wish we had signed up for the inexpensive Department of Aging transportation that could have transported my mom to and from the adult center. I guess I always worried that they might not take her to the right place,

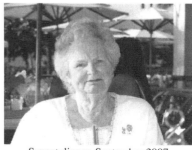
Sunset dinner, September 2007

and I couldn't bear the thought of her being lost. I had heard a few stories about people getting lost while being transported but having that resource handy on occasion could have been useful. Months after Mom's arrival the doctor suggested we get a handicapped parking pass, which we really needed with the pain Mom had in her legs from the peripheral artery disease. We should have gotten that sooner, as well as keeping a wheelchair at hand.

Once the "writing is on the wall," you must stop thinking in temporary terms! Get documents drawn up; contact the Department of Aging to see what services they offer; hire in home help; check out adult day centers; and get a handicap parking pass. Even if your situation is temporary, these simple things may be of help to you.

 HELPFUL HINTS

Documents you will need: Will, POA- Power of Attorney, Living Will, HIPAA-Health Insurance Portability and Accountability Act, EMS & DNR- Emergency Medical Services and Do not Resuscitate Medical Care Order. (see appendix)

Find a doctor or, more specifically, a geriatrician, who is a doctor who specializes in the health problems of the elderly.

Look around your home or place of caregiving for danger zones.

Stop in several adult day care centers to see which one may suit your loved one.

If you hire help to come into your home, get references from your doctor or friends as to what agency to use. Be sure background checks have been performed. Do not leave money, checkbooks, or valuables lying around.

Chapter 5
JUGGLING WORK & DAY CARE

Pete actually went to get Mom from the rehabilitation center in Maryland on a Wednesday night red eye flight arriving in Maryland on Thursday and returning to Hawaii on Saturday with her. This was a huge gift to me, as I was two weeks into a new school year and still establishing routines. I should have known that something was different when, after the long flight and time change from Maryland to Hawaii, Mom was up for going out to dinner rather than to bed early! However, Pete was beginning to see first hand the extent of the damage to her brain. During the long flight back, they were watching a feature film with a story line about a family member who is just diagnosed with dementia! Pete mumbled to a seat partner that, quite ironically, this was our story as well. The best part was when Mom announced she was bored with the movie and was going to get off the "bus." Pete told her she wouldn't be able to open the door without being tackled. When she asked why, he explained that they were in a plane over the Pacific. Boy, was she surprised with that answer!

We all felt that our three month rehabilitation project was going to be fun! After all, I was an educator with psychology and rehabilitation as my minors. Not yet knowing the very mild memory issues had been greatly exacerbated by the stroke, we thought this would be a breeze getting Mom back to one hundred percent. The neurologist said that there was an approximate 90-day window to recover from a stroke. This three month time frame is not an absolute in every case but rather a general guideline. What you have at three months is pretty much what you get, as usually not much more progress takes place after that time frame. But what I love most about the brain is that it can surprise doctors. A great doctor will tell you that we cannot fully understand the brain. Never underestimate the self-healing power of the brain.

At first it was such a novelty having Mom with us and doing everyday things such as grocery shopping, going to the beach, and even cooking together, which was not something we had usually done. The cooking together turned out to be not such a good idea. I remember "we" were making stuffed green peppers. She nearly cut her finger off trying to hollow out the green pepper! That was the last time we cooked together.

There was no way to ease Mom into going to the adult day care center. She thought that she could stay at our house all day, but we were concerned that she was at risk to have another stroke or perhaps a heart attack. We had no idea how badly her brain had been affected by the stroke- just yet. Our family was still in "rehab mode." We insisted she go to the center during our work hours. We did briefly introduce her to Nora on the way back from the airport so she could informally assess her, as, I guess, not everyone is accurately portrayed on the application by family! Nora was kind enough to meet us on Sunday when they were closed so Mom could begin Monday morning.

Pete took her there that first day instead of me so that if she had objections, I would not be late for a class full of fourth graders. I remember having my phone on my desk, half expecting a phone call. Thank God, my school and the adult center were only a block away from each other. I went to get her just as soon as my teaching day was done, anxious to see how things went, like an anxious mother going to get her child after the first day of school. To everyone's delight, she had enjoyed herself and made friends easily...perhaps too easily.

I am grateful that when all this happened to Mom that we were living in Hawaii. In the Hawaiian culture, elders are appreciated and revered, as in Asian cultures. Everyone was kind and accepting toward Mom, and she quickly blended in with the group. However, picture a room full of Asian and Pacific Islanders, and here comes the white girl with a huge dimply smile. Now also picture two groups of people within the center: highly able mentally but physically challenged people and those who need full care because they can't communicate or get out of a wheelchair. Well, the white gal was soon nicknamed "Little Miss Sunshine" to all who knew her. She came in with a smile very day, but perhaps the nickname started when she wore her bright yellow jogging suit. A few months later when she was still able to dress herself, I remember picking her up in that same suit, but she had the jacket off... but with no shirt on... just her see-through undershirt... yup, and NO BRA. Mom had joined the 60's "burn your bra" revolution in 1995. While on vacation in England, she stood behind a pub and wiggled out of her bra proclaiming she was done with bras! So maybe she was having a flashback!

As you can imagine, Little Miss Sunshine was quite popular with the men. A couple of them told me how beautiful she was with her fair skin, white hair, and dimples. She soon came home mentioning her "boyfriend" Ralph. We think one Ralph actually worked there, but her second boyfriend named Ralph was a volunteer. He would smuggle in candy bars for the diabetic Little Miss Sunshine - a definite no-no! But alas, that was the least of our concerns. They were caught kissing on more than one occasion, and Ralph was married! Well, needless to say, Mom got this volunteer fired with her flirtatious behavior!

To our great surprise, Mom settled into a daily routine

at the center. She loved the social interactions, and she kept us on our toes, referring to it as either going to "work", or "school." Some days she would tell us all about her "paperwork" for the day. She would tell us about how she would sit at her desk, do her "paperwork," and then file it. When we would send her in with her monthly payment fee, she would protest! Mom would say, "With all the paperwork I do, they should pay me!" Some days she would talk about "school" and all the things she would learn, such as the then - Presidential candidate Barack Obama was a "nice man" who came from Hawaii. Little Miss Sunshine had forgotten she was a diehard Republican!

The daily routines were great for mom. The center had bingo, arts and crafts, word games, dances, exercises, and, of course, naptime which was anytime for some people! Her favorite exercise was called "Pick the Mangoes," where the residents would reach their arms up in the air to pretend to pick a mango.

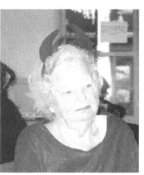
Halloween at the adult day care center, October, 2007

Mom regularly mentioned moving back to her condo in Annapolis. My brother Steve called weekly, and she would mention this to him. Believing us, but not quite knowing the extent of her dementia at first, he would encourage Mom to get her credit card, book a flight, take a cab to the airport, and return home! Of course, she could no longer do all those steps. And on those occasions when she would "whisper" to him over the phone that I was driving her nuts and she had to move back, he would empathize with her and agree by saying, "I wouldn't want to live with Luann either!"

Although we were physically and emotionally drained

40

juggling work and caring for Mom, we didn't know those two years were the very best of times. Although we were exhausted, she was with us, had a good place to spend her days, and was stimulated mentally, and it was our privilege to care for her. I should have appreciated each day more...and laughed more. My parents had sacrificed so much for my brother and me, and I was glad to be there when she needed it most.

 HELPFUL HINTS

If you are considering adult day centers, visit them without an appointment to see how they run when not expecting a visitor. That will not be a problem for the good centers. Ask about specific activities.

Compile a list of a few names of people who know your loved one and can be reached in case of an emergency. Put them on the emergency list at the center.

Find work/life balance and don't forget to take care of yourself. You can't properly take care of others if you are physically/mentally drained. Pete told me later that he used to feel guilty going for his much needed long weekend runs because he felt bad about leaving me with Mom. Then he began to put on weight and felt worse!

If you regularly attend a place of worship, continue to make time for it. Feeling overwhelmed at times, we became irregular attenders at church, which was not a good idea in hindsight.

I made copies of Mom's license and wrote COPY across the front and on the back listed all our contact information. Then I laminated them. I put one in her purse and coat pocket.

Keep a medicine list/doctor contact list with all caretakers/day care providers at all times. I also put a copy in Mom's purse.

Get yearly flu shots and the pneumonia vaccine as recommended by your geriatrician. Any ongoing cough should be checked for TB.

Statistically, caregivers over time can lose several promotions at work. I believe that others who have not chosen to caregive in their own family situation can be resentful if you are caregiving. I have seen this with my friends. They may feel left out in making decisions or they are just too far away to help. Perhaps they are jealous of the close relationship developing with your spouse or children if you caregive in your home. Others may be suspicious of how you are spending your family member's money, so keep detailed records and receipts. Or, perhaps, they just feel guilty for not being there to help more.

Chapter 6
FAKING IT & LOSING THINGS

In the early stages of dementia, when hindsight is 20/20, your loved one may try to fake answers to direct questions to which they do not know the answer. Also, they may show signs of misplacing things or have difficulty staying organized. I even found that Mom's closest friends were telling her, and eventually us, that something horrible was beginning to happen in her brain.

When Dr. Mark and others asked Mom a few questions from the Mini-Mental State Examination (MMSE)*, it was clear she was "faking it" in her replies. She was mild to moderately demented, so Mom would try her best to disguise her answer. For example, if she was asked how old she was, she would pause for a moment, then smile, flash her dimples and coyly respond, "Old enough to know better!" punctuated with a wink! Early in the disease she could remember the year she was born but couldn't process the math to figure out her age or perhaps couldn't remember the present year. When asked who the current president was, she would try the stalling decoy and say, "Oh, you know, um ..." and try to have you say the answer. She was a master at these techniques, but then Dr. Mark and I gave each other knowing glances. She was so resourceful that a hospitalist once noticed her "cheating" for answers! Mom was asked the date and year, and Dr. Stephanie noticed that her eyes were looking at the white board with the answers over her shoulders, you know, the dry erase board that lists the day, date, RN, and tech for the day. If that wasn't enough, Mom would try to glance at the newspaper on her tray to get answers to these questions.

My tidy mother was no longer quite as tidy, but she kept the "little messes" in closets or cupboards where they weren't seen. She began to claim she was losing things, which was not always true. Many of these things were imagined or misplaced rather than lost. I told you earlier about when she called to say she had lost her car in the parking lot, which was true, but she was calling me from home after having retrieved her car with assistance. We know from cleaning out her home that she did not lose two driver's licenses when she claimed the hospital had lost them, but they were neatly tucked away in a wallet in her dresser. On another occasion she emerged from a ladies room, claiming that she had washed her hands and washed a ring down the drain. We had not been with her all that day, but if she did wash one down the sink, we never figured out which one.

When Mom first came to live with us in Hawaii, she took pride in her appearance using makeup, combing her hair, and putting on her watch, rings, and earrings. Many a day we were looking for a lost earring, but they always turned up-except one pair of opal earrings. I suspect she gave that pair to a friend at the adult center. Over time, these things became less important, but while living with us, Mom always maintained her routine. When she moved into the assisted living home in Colorado, they suggested that we not leave any good jewelry there, so she just had her watch which, in her final months, was often worn upside down.

My favorite, the "lost purse episode," was when we were in Kmart shopping. She had gone to the ladies room. A little while later we asked where her purse was, and with hand gestures she claimed it must have been stolen. We retraced our steps, thinking she had laid it down somewhere; we looked in the ladies room. Yup, it was still hanging safe and sound on the back of the stall door where she had just used the toilet.

We gave Mom enough change at the beginning of each week to buy one soda each day while living with us and attending the center. We put it in a little change purse for her, but usually by Wednesday mom had no change left. I suspect she had more than one per day and perhaps bought some for friends. But Mom never forgot to bug us each day for her change. At least it was diet soda...I hope!

If you know your loved one's friends, they are a great resource regarding your loved one. I wish my mother's close friends had told us their concerns sooner. One of Mom's close friends stopped hanging out with her because of cancelled dates or not calling her friend back. At the time we thought it was my Mom's friend's issue, as she was several years older. We didn't know it was actually my mom's issue. Another close friend of Mom's started describing, "deer in the headlights" behavior by my mom while playing bridge. This was a huge sign, but we didn't put together all the symptoms until way too late. Mom had a history of Transient Ischemic Attacks, TIA's**, also known as 'mini strokes' in her medical history. Often a person can be engaged in something like a card game or talking when they stop for a moment, gaze off, and then continue the activity after several seconds. Sometimes this behavior can be mini-strokes, and if left untreated, it can lead to dementia.

Mom was never officially diagnosed with any particular type of dementia, but it seems in hindsight it was Vascular Dementia, VaD.*** While living in Hawaii, my dear friend Ann, a nurse, was a constant support to us. Ann and I had assumed that this was the form of dementia we were dealing with and that her decline would be gradual like stair steps. For many weeks our family would see no change but then suddenly a step down. Mom was dealing with dementia, but the stroke fast-forwarded her decline. She survived nearly three and a half years after the life-altering stroke. Mom had every symptom of Vascular Dementia: stroke, mini strokes, atherosclerosis, high blood pressure, diabetes, and atrial fibrillation (A-Fib). The only thing that didn't describe her was that Mom never had a heart attack and had quit smoking around 35 years ago. As her ailments grew, why didn't the doctors tell us about the road on which we were headed?

I was there in the hospital in 2002 when the neurologist came in to assess her. She had been having TIA's or mini strokes, and Mom had high blood pressure and diabetes. Why didn't the doctor tell me where this was most likely headed? Or why didn't the cardiologist, who added a pacemaker to regulate her heart due to A-Fib, which is another risk for stroke and knew her medical history, tell me the road we were on? And finally, why didn't the vascular surgeon, who had all this information, performed carotid artery surgery, and later put a cryogenic artery in her leg due to Peripheral Artery Disease (PAD)****
tell us to see a geriatrician? Perhaps a specialist, such as a geriatrician, would have overseen all Mom's meds and medical history and could have prevented the stroke by putting her back on blood thinners or recommended dementia drugs then? When the vascular surgeon did the leg surgery, I was her HIPAA representative. Why didn't he spell out the risks for me? Why didn't someone put all the pieces of this puzzle together? Why did it take me writing a book to figure this out for myself?

  HELPFUL HINTS

*MMSE- The Mini-Mental State Examination, an excellent barometer of whether one may be in early stages of dementia, can be found online. Copyright: M.

46

Folstein, S Folstein, P MCHugh. See example: enotes. tripod.com/MMSE.pdf

Drawing a clock can be another small part of a test for dementia. Patients will not be able to draw the numbers on the clock in the proper order or will more likely put the numbers all on one side of the clock.

**TIA's-Transient Ischemic Attacks - also known as 'mini strokes'

***VaD- Vascular Dementia, according to the Mayo Clinic, is caused by conditions that damage blood vessels which reduce the supply of nutrition and oxygen to the brain. This condition is often the result of stroke or a series of TIA'S. Other contributing factors include age, history of heart attack, atherosclerosis, high blood pressure, diabetes, smoking, and atrial fibrillation.

****PAD- Peripheral Artery Disease - Mayo Clinic describes as a circulatory problem in which narrowed arteries reduce the blood flow to limbs. It often may be a sign to more widespread fatty deposits (plaques) in arteries which can lead to atherosclerosis. This can cause reduced blood flow to the brain.

Minimize stuff for them to lose. They don't need access to all their jewelry or a full purse/wallet. Let your loved one have the important pieces (or copies of things) but let them have less to lose.

My mom always asked to carry her credit card although she had no need to use it. Save the preapproved plastic credit card looking items that come in the mail and give them one of those instead.

Chapter 7
CHILDLIKE HONESTY

Children are born honest. They say what they think and think what they say. At some point, parents teach their children to be dishonest...or perhaps to hold back from speaking aloud their honest thoughts. You know, when you have them in a public setting, and they meet one of your friends and say, "You're fat." Or perhaps you go to someone's home for dinner and your child announces, "Your house is really messy." We've all had those embarrassing moments with children because of their honesty. And then begin the "lessons" with our children about how we should only say "nice" things aloud. As Art Linkletter would say on his TV show where he asked kids random questions, "Kids Say the Darndest Things!"

Well, people with dementia, at some point, return to this childlike honesty, and you cannot teach them to hold back! Sometimes the problem was that Mom would say such comments, thinking she was whispering, but she wasn't! Now, she was also hard of hearing, but that made it even more fun to talk about her, in front of her, at times! (This was another survival technique for our family!) And her quite loud "whispered" comments came at the most awkward times, like the time we were getting our nails done, and she asked an attractive older woman if that was her grandchild with her. She had not noticed the fact that the child was calling the woman "Mommy." Or the time she asked who that "fat man" in the doorway of her hospital room was, who happened to be her nurse. Another time I routinely colored my hair, and it may have been a bit redder than normal, but she rarely noticed such details anymore. However, this time she said, "What did you do to your hair?" I just glared at her as she went on to say, "I may not know much, but I know that you're not a redhead!" My family enjoyed that comment!

As another part of our family coping mechanism, we liked to tell Mom tall tales or kid with her about her lack of observation. For a woman who used to notice every detail, this took some getting used to. Our son Peter had come out for Jess's graduation from the University of Hawaii in May of 2009. At this point we rented a wheelchair to get Mom to the event because the walking would have been too much. We all stayed in a hotel downtown the night before graduation to avoid traffic that morning, as Oahu has only three highways! Mom was exhausted and slept through most of the ceremony. The next day as Peter was preparing to return to Massachusetts, Mom asked how he was getting home, and by this time Peter had caught on to our antics. He told her how he had rented a car but it was a long drive and that he was concerned about driving tired. She asked, "Can you fly?", but Peter told her it was too expensive. So they agreed that he would take a bus from Hawaii to Massachusetts and she gladly gave him some bus money! I guess it wasn't a good brain day...

When we moved from Hawaii to Colorado in July of 2009, Mom moved to an assisted living home. We toyed with Mom about Joe - her favorite friend there. He was, indeed, a good looking, intelligent, kind gentleman. In fact, at first we thought Joe worked there because he was always helping in the dining room and kitchen. We would tease her about her close friendship with Joe. It was sweet, and they looked out for one another. We would tease her about perhaps having a "cuddle" with Joe, but she said he had a "girlfriend." So, with that, Jessica said, "You know what they say, 'Once you go black, you never go back'." Then Mom slightly annoyingly replied, "I don't know what you're talking about." Jess responded, "Joe is black." She looked at me and then Pete as he nodded in agreement. (He was the only person she believed anymore.) Suddenly she said loudly, "He's black?" And she continued to mutter softly, "No, he's not…" Indeed, Joe was black, but it didn't matter to anyone, and Mom didn't believe us anyway! What made us chuckle was that she never noticed! In many ways it was a very happy world she now lived in with not a care in the world!

On another occasion Pete took Mom to church when I was visiting Jessica for her birthday while she was still living in Hawaii in May of 2010. She would often cat nap in church but then tell us how much she enjoyed it! But on this occasion the pastor during his sermon was recognizing the importance of family. He asked parents to stand and be recognized, and then he asked grandparents. Mom, attempting to follow along, hollered out, "Now what do you want us to do?" Those people sitting nearby got a chuckle. Thank God, I was not there because I don't think I would be laughing just then! Well, at least she was trying to follow along!

When Mom needed a perm while living in Colorado, I would take her to my hairdresser to get that done rather than to the woman who did her hair weekly at her assisted living home. We would make it an outing which often included going to lunch. Thankfully, my hairdresser Karen was familiar with this horrible disease. She was perfect for Mom and would go along with whatever Mom had to say! The first time they met, she asked Karen, "Am I getting a perm? Karen told her she was, and then Mom replied, "I'm just visiting here, so I don't know why I couldn't get this done at home!" But Karen just played along. On another occasion, Jessica took her to Karen for a perm, and I met up with them there. Jess had just moved to Colorado in September of 2010 and didn't know Karen or her great sense of humor. So, when Mom decided she was done getting the perm or she would "pinch Karen's tits" among other rude comments, Jess started to slump down in the chair wishing to be invisible, but then approached Mom and told her in no uncertain terms to cooperate. She reminded her that Karen was almost done and we would be going out for lunch and sat back down. She filled me in on Mom's bad behavior when I arrived. Still wishing to have the perm over with, we overheard her tell Karen, "If I have to sit through this, it better be a steak dinner not just lunch!"

Yes, there were plenty of embarrassing moments.... many of which took place in restaurants. Mom was forgetting
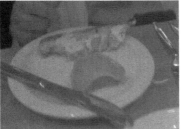
things such as how to cut her food or even eat it. She had no clue how to eat corn on the cob anymore. And napkins... well, they served two functions now! Yup, wiping one's mouth and blowing one's nose! On one occasion she gently placed her upper dentures on her bread plate, declaring that it was easier to chew the bread and crust without them!

Mom thought it was easier to chew the bread without teeth....

Since Mom was a little hard of hearing, it was easy to talk softly about her in front of her! It even got to the point that while saying grace as we gathered for dinner, we would beg the Good Lord to take her to her heavenly home, of course, in His timing. We openly talked about the possibilities of her dying or helping to complete her "bucket list" even if we had to hire actors! This shocked Jessica's then boyfriend Landon whom she knew from the University of Hawaii. During Jessica's birthday dinner in 2009, while saying grace, we once again pleaded for the Good Lord to come for her, and I thought Landon was going to choke! As he got to know us, Mom, and this horrible disease, I think he understood our prayer.

Landon, being of Mexican descent, taught us a fun little car game he called, "Mexican Air Conditioning" he would play as a child. On really hot days he would close the windows, turn the heat up in his car, then shut it off and then open the windows. This would make the outside air seem cooler for a few brief moments. He suggested we try it one day as we were all in the car together. Mom would begin sweating and complaining, and we would pretend that it wasn't hot at all. Shameless, I know, but on one occasion it totally backfired on us! As we played the game, Mom never said a thing. Temperatures were rising, and we all began sweating, except Mom! She never even noticed the sweat literally dripping off Landon as he sat beside her. We never played the game again.

Our dear friend and neighbor in Hawaii, Diane, took care of Mom when all three of us had to leave the island on a couple of occasions. Mom thought it was ridiculous to

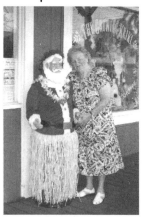

Mom always
"believed" in Santa

have someone come and stay with her. After all, she could get herself to the adult day care center and go to the store, etc. When we told her she didn't have a car and no longer drove, she then agreed to let Diane drive her! This is where "creative" answers came in, and we encouraged Diane to do so. (I'm sure God understood our creativity and that it wasn't really considered lying.) So, one night Mom insisted that she would be fine alone and Diane could pick her up the next morning. Diane replied, "Oh, I know you'll be fine; it's Holly (our golden retriever) I'm worried about!" And that was why Diane would sleep over...to take care of Holly, of course!

My favorite embarrassing stories with Mom always

involved her love for men! She was a flirt until the day she died! Our internist in Hawaii, Dr. Mark was kind enough to take Mom on with his busy practice. Of course, we all thought it was just going to be for a few months. She loved to go see him as he was a very good looking, kind hearted middle aged man. He had a wonderful, reassuring way with his patients not to mention a great smile. One day he asked her to lie down so he could check her stomach. She replied, "Oh, that's what all the men say to me!" He blushed, and I just rolled my eyes. What else could I do? If it was a thought in her head, it came out her mouth with a lack of filters.

But she outdid herself at embarrassing him on another visit. Dr. Mark had to tell her about a concern he had seen on her mammogram. After a routine mammogram, another one was needed because of something they had seen on her X-ray. He sweetly told her this as I was standing just behind his left shoulder. I saw her face fall. She must have remembered how her sister, Lil, had died of breast cancer. I knew I had to lighten the moment so I shrugged my shoulders and with hand motions exclaimed, "You have to die of something; it may as well be breast cancer!" She looked deeply into my eyes, then Dr. Mark's and simply stated, "I had hoped to die in bed with a man." I thought I would die when she said that, but poor Dr. Mark grinned shyly while turning the color of a tomato! I know he admired how we cared for Mom. He would often say that Mom was doing so well because of our loving care. And we admired how he still loved his work and truly cared for each of his patients after many years of doctoring.

We had many coping mechanisms in caretaking. It was crucial to keep well rested, eat well, squeeze in time for ourselves, and laugh a lot! So, we often competed, somewhat, in who could tell Mom the most convincing nonsensical story. It was great! One of us would start the story, and we would all add to it as we went along! It was actually a great gauge of where her brain was that day because with dementia there can be great fluctuation, especially in the presence of infection. Any infection makes dementia temporarily worse.

HELPFUL HINTS

Any infection, such as, urinary tract infections, temporarily increase the dementia. We knew Mom was starting one before she did. The urine smell was strong, and her dementia was worse.

The "childlike honesty" is just simply being honest, and while embarrassing at time, try not to be too embarrassed because most people will understand.

Telling "tall tales" is a useful coping mechanism. The first few months that Mom lived with us, she often argued about moving back to Annapolis. We didn't know at that point how useful a tall tale could have been. For example, we could have told her the condo was damaged in a tornado and was being repaired!

Laughter lowers your blood pressure, so laugh often.

Chapter 8
THE SIMPLE THINGS IN LIFE

The simple truth about dementia is that it changes certain aspects of one's personality. These changes can be for better or worse. For Mom, the changes were better. She had been a high strung, goal oriented worrier! I guess this process of change began with the beginning of the dementia during 2003; however, the stroke in 2007 permanently affected her brain. She physically recovered from the full left side stroke. It was, in fact, remarkable how much the clot busting, tPA drug (Ch. 1) helped her. What we hadn't known was that her mild dementia was now moderate, a permanent change from the stroke, no matter how much we stimulated her brain during the approximately 90 day window of recovery that the neurologist had described.

When Mom came to live with us, Dr. Mark lowered her blood pressure medicine by half. Life had fewer worries and concerns. She had a more go-with-the-flow attitude.

Eating dinner out had always been one of her favorite things, but now she really enjoyed restaurants, especially the dinners near our home in Hawaii where we could sit and see the ocean and sunset. In fact, we were on a first name basis with the waiters. A hot dog dinner with ice tea was now one of her absolute favorite choices. The newly opened Costco on the island was another favorite hot dog hangout. Mom, who had traveled the world, was incredibly happy eating anywhere. She continued to enjoy the company of others and continued one of her favorite past times, people watching.

Suddenly, Mom really enjoyed the simple things in life. She had always been difficult to buy gifts for because she had the things she wanted. And she was a firm believer in shopping to lift one's spirits. So, giving her gifts when she was with us during those last three years was fun! She delighted in anything you gave her and had a sense of childlike wonder. During Christmas she opened things slowly because she was still enjoying the item opened previously. Mom would begin to open the next gift and sometimes stop and pick up the last one opened to examine it more closely. And when we would hand her another gift, she would say, "For me?" with great surprise in her voice. In fact, we could rewrap gifts from last year, and she would enjoy them as if it were her first time seeing them!

Mom was never a nature or animal lover so, understandably, animals were not her thing. However, in her demented state she loved our dog Holly. Unfortunately, Holly, for me was like looking in a mirror because Holly could read my emotions so easily. Holly was super sensitive to the moods in our home. Some days she would greet me at the door, take one look at the frustration in my face already there from the short ride home, and go off in a corner to hide. Mom would say to Holly at least 20 times per day, "Holly, good dog." I longed to hear, just once, "Luann, good daughter," but, alas, I never did. She often spoke about what a good man Pete was and what wonderful children I had. After a couple of years, Mom even liked our cat Lizzie! She had always hated cats, a phobia passed along from her mother who was nicknamed Kitty because of her fear of cats.

One day after we had moved to Colorado, we picked Mom up from her assisted living home and instead of going out to dinner, we had picked up Subway subs, fresh cookies, and her favorite soda. It was a beautiful, warm summer's evening, so we took Mom to a nearby park with picnic tables. Because sub sandwiches were always hard for her false teeth, we cut it in small pieces, and she never complained. She was going for the prize...the cookie! Normally, she would have not enjoyed such an outing, but instead she marveled in the beautiful evening and the ducks and ducklings swimming in the nearby pond. We stayed until nearly sunset, and I will always treasure that night. This is also because her legs gave out on a couple of large steps she couldn't maneuver as we headed to the car, and

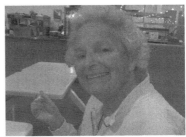

Mom wearing the "Little Miss Sunshine" outfit having a hotdog dinner.

I still have the pictures of Pete trying to hoist her like a crane in order to get her back up! Priceless.

Over the three years, Mom often spoke of loved ones and sometimes forgot people were dead. They came to her in her dreams. On one particular evening Pete and I had run a quick errand and returned to find Mom watching TV and sobbing. We asked her what was wrong and she explained that she "didn't know" where her mother was. When we told her that she died years ago, she got hysterical. She asked, "What?" in a whining, disbelieving voice then followed by, "Was I there?" Then she looked at Pete and said, "Were we married then?" Now Pete, who had the patience of Job, had a look of horror flash across his face. Then he told her in a booming voice while shaking his head and waiving a finger gesturing 'us,' "WE WERE NEVER MARRIED!" Mom seemed disappointed and appeared to not fully believe Pete or understand his reaction. However, some of her behaviors began to make sense...the way she would greet him after work, pet his arm, and occasionally grab his butt! She thought they were married and perhaps there were times Mom was treating me as "the other woman!" We explained that she had been vacationing in Florida when her mother passed, but reassured her that she had attended the funeral.

On another occasion, she told me she dreamed about my very conservative, Archie Bunker-type dad and said she dreamed he had a ponytail! I asked her how he looked, and she said, "Good!" Mom and Dad had separated late in life but stayed in constant touch. My father even reached out and called her in the last moments of his life, but, unfortunately, Mom was not there to receive the call. Mom only recalled the best times that they shared over 40 years of marriage.

Several months before Mom died, she wanted to purchase a Mother's Day card for her mom who had died over 25 years ago. In hindsight, what would have been the harm in purchasing a card and asking her to dictate the message she wanted written in the card? I missed out on a profound opportunity. Instead, I hurt her with the truth that she didn't need to hear.

Mom liked to recall stories about her childhood regularly. In Mom's recollection she was Cinderella, and her sister, Lillian, who was often sick, got away with fewer chores. I am sure this was somewhat of an exaggeration. Mom often spoke of her brother Vern with whom she loved to attend square dances. He would call the square dance and also played in the band. Mom also recalled how she was paid a dollar per game to keep score for his baseball team. She loved and admired her mother, who raised three children single-handedly during the 1930's, and rarely spoke of her father who had left the family when she was young.

When we would visit Mom at her assisted living home in Colorado, she was always so excited to see us. It was as if we were her long lost relatives whom she hadn't seen in years. She would give me one of those tight lingering hugs around my neck and a kiss on the cheek, and I know I must have been rolling my eyes. While we were a moderately affectionate family, this type of greeting was way over the top! Now that she is gone, I would give anything for one of those "over the top" hugs.

Mom was truly happy with the simplest things in life. Seize those moments and enjoy them.

 HELPFUL HINTS

Maybe I was wrong to always tell her that the loved ones she often dreamed about were dead. I guess I hadn't realized the extent of the disease, and I could have softened my responses or even assured her she would be seeing them in some vague response.

Attempt to have a more go with the flow attitude as well. Go with what they need to do or hear. I am convinced that God honors this sort of white lie in such situations.

Caregiving can drain your budget, so purchase simple, usable gifts or re-gift.

Chapter 9
SAFETY & WANDERING

Our first wandering experience happened on a vacation to Hawaii during Christmas break 2003, when we weren't even aware that Mom was in the early stage of dementia. We took this trip to show our son Peter, Jess, and Mom the area where we would be moving the following July. Mom happily agreed to join us on that vacation, as she had been to Hawaii several times before, and it was her favorite place on earth!

One morning after breakfast, we decided to run a quick errand. We told Mom we would be back shortly. Still in her P.J.'s, she seemed in no hurry to go anywhere quickly so we left her at the hotel. When we returned, she was nowhere to be found! She was not in the room or anywhere in the hotel, and no note was left. We were debating calling the police and local hospitals when she finally returned several hours later. We were beside ourselves, thinking a medical emergency had taken place or worse, but she seemed truly confused by our concern. We asked in a firm tone where she had been. She explained that she had walked to The International Market Place and gone shopping which, other than flirting with men, was her favorite thing to do. It was a bit of a walk for someone with peripheral artery disease, which was amazing in itself, and in that she didn't get lost. If you haven't ever been to The International Market Place in Waikiki, it is a bargain shopper's delight! She took great pride in showing us all her "finds," still quite unaware of our concerns. We jokingly told her she was "grounded" for the rest of the trip and not allowed out of our sight. Yup, full circle- grounding my mother! It was a foreshadowing of things to come.

We were still in Hawaii on Christmas Eve so Mom, being

the "shouting" Methodist she called herself, found
a church for us to attend that evening. We looked
forward to the candlelight service but upon our arrival
realized that the service was being spoken in Korean!
All five of us piled back into the car, and son Peter
dutifully checked the newspaper and map of downtown
simultaneously-smart boy. He announced that he had
found a Baptist Church in the vicinity. So, Pete followed
Peter's directions, but before having this bunch get out
again, he ran in to check out the church. He ran back
to the car only to disappoint us with the news that the
service was being spoken in Vietnamese! It was now 7:00
p.m. and our options were limited on attending any service
at all. Just then, after studying the map, Peter excitedly
announced that he had found a Christian Church nearby
and with any luck at all we would only be a few minutes
late. It was our last hope.

We parked and all got out and, to our surprise, not only
was the service being spoken in English, there were seats!
We sat in the last row, not wanting to disturb others.
Of course, after all this driving around, Mom had to use
the bathroom. I went with her, not wanting to "lose"
her again, and asked a nearby woman where it was. She
took us to the bathroom and waited with us. I guessed
that was because there was only one bathroom in the
building. The bathroom was a stall-like structure inside
the pastor's study. We could see each other's feet from
under the door as we took turns using the toilet. Mom
was a great communicator with her eyes and after using
the bathroom gave me the "Would you believe?" look that
started her grinning.

We were escorted back to our seats by the somewhat
strange lady who seemed distrustful of us. It didn't
take Jess and me too long to realize there was a unique
aspect to this church. We elbowed Peter and Mom, then

61

whispered that Pete and I were the only heterosexual couple/family there! When Mom realized that it was true, she couldn't stop chuckling softly. At that point Pete, my serious husband, was trying to follow the sermon and a bit clueless to the demographics of the congregation, gave us an annoying "Shh" signal! Now Peter, Jess, and I were losing it at the sight of Mom who was never subtle. Mom was trying to be quiet with her hands and head resting on her cane, which was between her legs, and staring at the floor. However, it didn't help because Mom got a case of the giggles as her entire body shook almost silently with laughter. We all tried to focus on the Christmas story while visiting this congregation. Strange though, the pastor announced a hymn sing along and refreshments after the service, but no one greeted us or encouraged us to stay after the service. At least we didn't lose her that night. Months later I recalled that story and route to Jessica's University of Hawaii advisor who was nearly blind and whose husband was a pastor. She knew exactly where we had been: the Korean Methodist Church, the Vietnamese Baptist Church and The First Christian Church, and she smiled as she noted that we attended the gay church.

There were many adventures with Sophie and Kasey, Jess's two closest girlfriends from the University of Hawaii. The first time Pete, Mom, and I met them was after Mom had just been released from the hospital in September of 2008, after a bout with cellulitis.* The three of us were anxious to meet Jess's new friends so we all met at a nearby restaurant. The girls didn't mind that Mom, coming directly from the hospital, was still sporting her hospital bracelet, robe, and slippers. She was happy to be going on an outing and bragged about her new "whistles," which were actually the ports to the central line of the IV. We had been instructed on how to give her IV antibiotics over the next week while at home.

Kasey and Sophie were dear friends who supported Jess and were a part of many of our adventures which often included wandering.

On one occasion Jess, Sophie, Mom, and I were shopping in Macy's. In recent years Mom had developed an aversion to escalators, so we took the elevator instead. We were all talking and realized too late that Mom had not stepped off the elevator with us. The elevator doors shut before we could grab her, and we frantically began to check all three floors, which took literally just minutes. We found her with some kind people helping her to look for us, and she was in the...men's department!

Sophie was always so kind and gentle with Mom, as was once again evident during a visit with us in August of 2009 just after we moved to Colorado. Sophie, Jess, Pete, and I went to visit Mom in her assisted living home and take her out to dinner. Sophie could see the

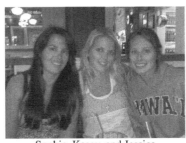

Sophie, Kasey, and Jessica

toll the disease was taking on Mom, as it had been just a few months since she last had seen her. Sophie lovingly walked with Mom arm in arm, chatting as girlfriends do. It was a beautiful sight, so I asked Sophie if she ever considered a career working with the elderly. She nervously replied, "You don't know what I'm thinking in my head!" So, even as I picture that beautiful image in my mind's eye, Sophie was telling me that working with the elderly was clearly not her comfort zone.

During a trip to Maui over Thanksgiving of 2008, Kasey joined our family. I knew the dementia was worsening because Mom no longer seemed to enjoy traveling because she missed the familiar. Traveling became difficult for her due to lack of routines. Kasey decided that Mom's reason for not joining us by the pool was that she "had to catch up on her paperwork" from "work" even while on vacation. We kept a close eye on her as we sat by the pool, not wanting to lose her again. We took a drive later that evening, and it was a beautiful evening. Unfortunately, someone had passed gas in the car which always evoked quite a reaction from Mom. So, to be sure of her typical over-reaction, Pete closed and locked the car windows. My Dad used to say, "Grin and bear the shame rather than bear the pain." It was in that moment that Mom disowned us. She swore to

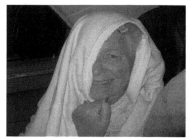

Mom's "gas mask"

Kasey that she didn't know us and was not part of our family. Furthermore, she tried to use her sweater as a gas mask. Laughter, the best medicine for stress!

During that same trip we had borrowed a wheelchair when we had to walk a lot, and we began "wheelchair races" with Mom in the chair. She was not a fan, but the more we could cause her hair to blow back, the harder we laughed. She begged her new friend Kasey for help, even asking her, "Kasey, help! Don't you want to be in my will?" But even in Mom's demise, she always remembered Jess's friends who were a part of her life during those two years in Hawaii. Sophie, Kasey, and Landon helped our family more than they will ever know.

Another wandering experience happened when Pete brought Mom with him to drop off my old X-rays, which I had forgotten, while I was having a routine mammogram. They, of course, needed them for comparison purposes. I waited for Pete to arrive. He parked the car at the entrance nearest the door to the office I was in. It was probably less than twenty feet away. He told Mom he would be right back and even left the keys in the car. I was done with my exam when Pete arrived, so we gave the staff my X-rays. We walked out together, and as I was walking with Pete to his car, Mom was nowhere in sight! After several minutes of frantically searching, we found her emerging from the ladies room. Again, she didn't understand that she had left a car with keys in it and disappeared on us. She was just simply using the bathroom.

On another day, exhausted and on my way home from school, I ran into Kmart to pick up my mom's prescriptions and told her I would be right back. She seemed to understand, and I quickly got the prescriptions and was walking through the store toward the exit. Suddenly, I saw this elderly woman wandering aimlessly in the store and after a double take realized it was Mom! I said, "You were supposed to stay in the car!" But you guessed it, she was looking for a bathroom. At least I didn't leave the keys in the car- I had learned that lesson. There were lots of bathroom stories, but what drove me craziest was every time we were driving on Interstate H1 and not near an exit, she would begin to think she might have to use a toilet. Then we would try to figure out the nearest exit or debate whether we could make it home in time. Fun...

One of the single most memorable, heartbreaking experiences was when Mom wandered from our condo in Hawaii one evening. We were all going to go to a movie one night, but something Mom ate didn't agree with her and gave her diarrhea. So, Pete helped her shower, and we put her PJ's on a bit early. She wanted to stay home and watch TV. So, at that point, we thought, what would the harm be, as she urged us to go. We rarely left her alone. We alerted our neighbor in the upstairs condo that we would be back within a couple of hours. Mom knew she could call upon Judy, our neighbor, so off we went. Upon driving into our neighborhood, Pete noticed something unusual and exclaimed, "Now look at that!" My night vision wasn't the best, and I thought he was referring to our indoor/outdoor cat Lizzy. Instead, he saw Mom, fully dressed, sporting her purse and attempting to enter a nearby building's upstairs condo. We, in fact, lived on the ground level. I'm not sure if I was more furious or deeply worried. Pete put the car in park and jumped out, running up the stairs and helping Mom back down asking, "What were you doing?" She replied that she was looking for us and that she...needed a bathroom. We reminded her that we had gone to a movie, and she remembered that but was "Looking for you!" This was one of the few times Pete was furious with her and upon returning home and getting her back in her PJ's, I don't recall her using the toilet. The truly amazing thing was that she dressed herself in one of her more challenging outfits! It was sort of a jacket style with only a sewn-in front shirt. It was the type that, when dressing herself, she would sometimes put the shirt part behind her back, which was always interesting. This occurred three months before our move, which, as we consulted with Dr. Mark, caused us to look for a secure facility for Mom in Colorado. Mom's wandering would only get worse, and he was wise.

In all seriousness, wandering will most likely become a problem at some point, and you should prepare for it. Also the biggest risk, other than wandering, is probably the risk of falling. Statistically, most elderly people with a broken hip requiring surgery do not survive longer than two years after the hip is repaired. I know this from when my dad had a broken hip in 2002. Another concern is fire, whether from the stove or microwave or perhaps scalding water, which is why constant companionship is essential. Stop and look and around your home for dangerous situations if your loved one lives with you. Area carpets which can slip should be removed. Make sure your loved one always wear shoes or slippers with good traction. A shower where you have to step into a tub is extremely dangerous. The first night Mom came to live with us, Jess and I both helped Mom in and out of the shower. She nearly pulled the two of us down. It then became Pete's job to help her in and out of the shower, which was a true labor of love.

Wherever you choose for your loved one to live with you in your home, or whether some other place, LOOK AROUND. Common sense safety factors are important.

HELPFUL HINTS

*Cellulitis is a bacterial infection, usually strep or staph, obtained through an opening in the skin such as a cut or even an insect bite which spreads to deeper tissues. People with weak immune systems, diabetes, and peripheral arterial disease are particularly susceptible. The infected area can be warm, red, and tender. Fever and chills may follow. Left untreated, it can lead to death.

Remove things that clutter pathways and area carpets that could cause falling.

Assist with showering to prevent scalding or falling. Make sure the shower has a slip proof surface or buy one. Adjust the temperature of your water heater if necessary.

If you have a gas stove, you may have to find some way to cover the controls. It's like making your home safe for a toddler again. It only takes a moment for an accident, and no one can watch a loved one every single moment.

Keep ID with your loved one in a wallet, purse, coat, etc. I made several copies of the front of her license, wrote "Copy" across the front and our contact information on the back. I laminated multiple copies and always had one or more with Mom.

Purchase door alarms to alert you if your loved one leaves your home or put bells on the doorknob.

I once was told this tip but didn't try it: put a large mirror on all exit doors. Demented people see the reflection but don't know it's a door. Additionally, a securely placed round, black area carpet at the exit doors can fool your loved one into thinking it is water.

Chapter 10
FULL CIRCLE

When you have the realization that you have become the "parent" to your parent, it is a very strange feeling. It's almost as though you have been suddenly orphaned or as if your parent were dead. But Mom still had a few powerful parenting moments left in her.

The most memorable moment was one disappointing day in teaching. I came home saddened by what a student had written concerning me. The weird part was a student whom I had poured my heart into had written something rude about me, only to get another student into trouble! In fact, he signed someone else's name and hadn't meant the comment to be true at all. I went to bed early that night feeling tired and sad. Mom was getting ready for bed, too, but asked Pete if it was all right for her to go in and speak with me. She came in and sat on the side of the bed. She rubbed my arm and spoke sweetly. She went on about how lucky my students were to have a teacher who cared as much as I did about her students and worked so hard. Additionally, she went on to talk about all the little lives I had touched over my many years of teaching and not to worry over one small incident. It was an incredible moment! It was one of those very last parenting moments that I will always treasure. Heck, it was actually all worth it, just to be a daughter once again...and have a mom.

Nowadays, things were different. Not only was I her HIPAA representative, but a few months down the road, I would also have a Power of Attorney over her affairs. We had had a role reversal. I had signed the documents for the adult day care as her guardian. I had to sign permission slips for her field trips at the adult center.

One such field trip took place a few months after her arrival. A few of the residents were going to a mall. I made sure to have Mom's "fake" ID on her with all of our phone numbers. However, this demented lady thought she should have her credit card with her to do a little Christmas shopping! This was a dangerous situation for sure! We got around that request by giving her around $20 in cash. When she returned, most of her cash had been spent on sweets, and she had a few cookies left to show for it. Mom was such a sneaky little diabetic!

Another outing involved a field trip to see the movie, Mamma Mia, which Mom had seen on Broadway. She was a well read and traveled lady. When she got home and we were just making dinner conversation, we asked her how she liked the movie. She replied, "Oh, it was OK," with a broad dimply grin. So, Pete and I glanced at one another and went on to ask her what the movie was about. Imagine our surprise to learn the movie was about a traveling salesman and a young girl whom he dated and she didn't really like him but he really liked her... "It was all right," she told us as she faked the storyline somewhat!

Another aspect of this full circle of life was helping put her clothes out the night before "work" or "school." She initially had little trouble getting some breakfast, taking the pills set out for her, and getting dressed. At the end of our two years in Hawaii, this progressed to helping her with all her morning tasks. She could no longer dress herself in a reasonable amount of time, and sometimes we discovered it too late. Pete would then have to drop her off on his way to work, making him a few minutes later than usual. At least he was on flex time, enabling him to work later as needed. As I've said before, I could not be late for my lively fourth graders! The progression of the disease was gradual but a downward slope.

Pete could always convince Mom to do anything because, as she told people at the center, I was the bitch and Pete could do no wrong. Except one day, he had to tell her that because she was taking a particular medicine (among countless other reasons), she could no longer drive. A huge debate/argument ensued, and she was not going to surrender her license! That is until I got home to finish the conversation-which wasn't a conversation at all. We had applied for a Maryland state ID card, as her license was due for renewal, and she still owned property there. We thought we could possibly return there to live in her home and continue caring for her. So, when I got home and Pete had given me the heads-up on the debate they were having, I simply stomped over, raised my voice, glared at her and demanded, "Sign it!" I guess I was the stricter "parent." And she signed it, and we never spoke about driving again.

The last few months in Hawaii, Mom was not always agreeable with us or others at the center. We began to pray that God would take her home before the disease worsened or, God forbid, the peripheral artery disease worsened and caused a leg to be amputated. This was her worst nightmare! She had had relatives who, years ago, had limbs amputated due to diabetes.

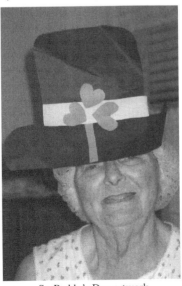

Probably the most interesting part of parenting my parent was figuring out what to do with all the artwork she created and brought home. I did what all parents do, I proudly displayed her pictures, newsletters, and "work" on the refrigerator.

St. Paddy's Day artwork

I still have the orange, fabric covered, toilet paper pumpkin she made. But, as I am of Irish descent, my favorite project was when she came out of the center wearing a St. Patrick's Day Hat, upside-down! Priceless. It looked like the same pattern as the fireman hats kids make in school only green and decorated for St. Patrick's Day. However, the upside-down way of sporting it had her looking a bit like a drunken Irishman!

I know that Jess, Pete, and I all had our own conversations with God about this horrible disease and why we were given the responsibility/burden/honor to care for her. But one thing we all knew was that there are no "ifs" in God's world. After all, she was sent to the "wrong" hospital, put on life support by "mistake" and was alive to tell the story-if she remembered it! No, there were lessons about unconditional love, patience, and compassion for us to learn. They were character building, difficult days and years for us.

HELPFUL HINTS

There is no preparation for when the day comes to parent a loved one. You finally recognize it: it just happens one day when you least expect it.

As mentioned before, keep plenty of ID/contact information and a list of medications with your loved one and yourself.

Go with whatever tall tale your loved one tells you in regard to their daily experiences. Telling tall tales goes both ways. Don't worry about being right!

Chapter 11
NETWORK OF FRIENDS & ANGELS

Psalm 91:11 tells us, "For he will command his angels concerning you to guard you in all your ways."

I don't think about angels on a daily basis, but I believe they exist. The Bible tells us that angels literally sometimes take on human form for a divine purpose and once that purpose is complete, they return to heaven.

Hebrews 13:2 says: "Do not forget to entertain strangers, for by so doing some people have entertained angels without knowing it."

Sometimes I really think I may have encountered angels while our family cared for Mom and other times perhaps angelic-like human beings. It is so important to have a support group of angelic type friends who know your loved one and whom you can count upon when needed.

In December 2006 I had to get back to Maryland from Hawaii in a hurry because Mom had not been feeling well, called an ambulance and, because the nearest hospital ER was too full, was sent to another hospital in Baltimore. This hospital had absolutely no records on Mom. As doctors tried to assess Mom, they must have gotten my phone number from her purse. I remembered the ER doctor calling me while I was shopping in Kmart and asking me all her medicines and medical conditions. As her HIPAA representative, I gave him my permission and pleaded with him to get her medical records from her local hospital, as she was taking approximately 13 different prescriptions at that time and had a complicated health history. The ER doctor said Mom had had a seizure, which I later realized had probably been brought on by diabetic shock, as she hadn't eaten for hours. Subsequently, Mom was put on life support via intubation to maintain an open airway and tubal feeding. This was against her wishes, but the hospital had no records.

We typically flew on one particular airline, and I had a friend named Nancy who worked for them. I knew Nancy because her son was in my fourth grade class. Between Nancy and Pete, they had me out on the first available flight the next morning. I solemnly boarded the plane thinking of leaving my students behind with a substitute but with the very sobering thought that I might not make it to Maryland in time or that I would be the one to take her off life support, according to her wishes. Just then I saw a familiar face. It was Margaret, our church pianist, who was also a flight attendant. It was so nice to see her on that flight, knowing that she was praying for me and pampering me all the way there. Peter picked me up from the airport as he had just so happened to be doing business in Baltimore rather than Massachusetts - his company's home base.

I often pondered Mom going to the Baltimore hospital rather than the one in her town because the ER was "too full." Mom's own hospital under the same circumstances would not have given her life support because her documents and wishes were scanned into their computer system. So, Mom ended up living another four years, almost to the day. Our family thinks that perhaps those additional years of life were for us to learn life lessons regarding the power of love and family. Angels, God, someone had their hand on all those details that day when her neighborhood hospital was "too full."

On another occasion we were eating at one of our favorite restaurants in Hawaii in 2007. Mom hadn't been living with us that long yet, and she was moderately

74

demented though continent. We all knew of Mom's diet restrictions: limit sugar and nothing made with milk. Milk products triggered her lactose intolerance, which, in turn, caused sudden and severe diarrhea because she also had ulcerated colitis. It seemed simple enough. However, on this particular evening, Mom had ordered a somewhat spicy pasta dish. This was our first and last encounter with spicy foods. After dinner, I was about to use the ladies room before we left. Mom inquired, "Are we going right home?" which was a fair enough question. Our family always has a way of getting sidetracked on outings and making stops at random places! I replied, "Yes" and she thought for a moment and then decided to go to the bathroom "just in case."

I had already gone ahead, and she was following behind me. I was tending to "my personal business" in the ladies room when I heard my mom crying and sobbing in the stall next to me. Actually, I could SMELL her before I heard her! The spicy food had caused the sudden onset of diarrhea with the worst stench I have ever smelled in my entire life. I quickly called Pete on my cell phone while I was still using the toilet. I exclaimed that I needed help now and hung up! By the time I was able to assist her, the diarrhea had already dripped down her legs and into her shoes. The smell was so strong my eyes were actually watering. Pete, from my brief phone conversation, thought Mom may have stroked again or that something worse may have happened. He ran to the ladies room with Jessica following closely behind. Pete slipped in her trail but not knowing that it was Mom's "stuff," yelled at a restaurant worker to "get that mess cleaned up" before someone really got hurt. He thought it was a food spill.

As Jess began to help, I had to leave the immediate scene because I literally felt sick. Pete and I concentrated on cleaning up her trail leading up to and

75

into the bathroom. It was then that we may have met an actual angel or at least an angelic human being. As several customers came upon this scene and chose not to use the ladies room, a beautiful young woman named Kristy, chose to come and help. She surveyed the chaos and said, "Can I help?" I looked and blinked in disbelief. She replied, "I do this for my work" referring to the fact that she worked in some kind of setting with the elderly and was used to poop messes. I don't care how used to poop she was, this was the worst ever! Kristy proceeded to go into the stall and help Jess with Mom. She left for a brief moment to go to her car where she just so happened to have a spare adult diaper, towel, and pair of her father's gym shorts! We had Mom and the floor cleaned up in no time, and Kristy returned to finish her meal with her husband and young daughter. We ushered Mom out a side door because she was crying and so embarrassed, not to mention she still reeked of eye-watering pooh stench.

As Jess and Mom briefly waited for us in the car, we apologized to the manager for the mess and paid for Kristy's family's meal. I somehow had the wherewithal to ask her husband for their address so I could wash and return the shorts. A week or so later I sent Kristy a note, gift card, the washed shorts, and a new pair of shorts as well. I think the package arrived, but I never heard from her or saw her again. Angel?

Another day I stopped on the way home from teaching to exercise as usual, or I would be too tired to do it later. Mom would often come inside either to just watch those working out or work on her crossword puzzles. One day Mom decided to wait in the car just outside the facility so she could people watch, a favorite pastime. I felt that she could find me as she had been there many times before and I was only going to be about 30 minutes or so.

76

After I finished and got in the car, Mom told me how she had been just fine and enjoyed sitting in the convertible as the weather was perfect. I noticed Mom had a bottle of water. I asked her where she got it from and she replied, "Some nice lady gave it to me." I found this interesting that some random woman noticed her sitting in the car and gave her water. Again, I thought perhaps Mom had encountered an angel.

Lisa, Mom's hairdresser in Hawaii, was another angel to us. She owned the hair salon, and Lisa knew how to do an old fashioned wash and set for a reasonable price. Lisa always made us feel welcome as we were often the only non-local people in her shop. Lisa loved our family, has deep faith in God, and remains a family friend to this day.

We had a wonderful group of friends who helped to support us, but the ones who always showed up when we needed them most and sometimes without even calling them were Jim and Diane. Diane would stay with Mom if we needed to travel off island, watch our pets, take Mom for a spin on their golf cart, or pick Mom up from the adult center as emergencies arose. On one particular occasion while we were off island, Diane had to call our friends, Bernie and Mike, to help with Mom's evening insulin. So, Mike willingly took the 15 minute drive, and as he arrived, found Mom tired and in bed already. With the room dimly lit, Mom couldn't resist the opportunity to engage this "nice man" in conversation. She asked, "Are you the doctor?" while reaching to pet his arm? And Mike couldn't resist saying, "No, but I play one [doctor] on TV," stolen from the character Joey on the FRIENDS show. I don't think she quite got the joke but

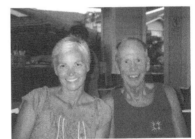
Diane and Jim

flashed a broad dimply, flirty smile.

We couldn't have made the move to Colorado without Jim and Diane, especially after Pete's motorcycle accident 10 days before our scheduled move. He totaled his motorcycle after a van stopped suddenly on Interstate H1, which gave him an unexpected ride to Shock Trauma at Queen's Hospital. Due to a broken leg, collar bone, ribs and fingers, I spent long days at the hospital with him. Thankfully, school was out for the summer. Diane or Jim would pick Mom up from the center and feed her dinner. After four days in the hospital Pete came home, Jim and Diane still offered to pick up Mom and give her dinner as we got organized for the move! They were always there when we truly needed them most. How was it that they always knew when we needed them?

And, how is it our old friend Diane from Colorado had a sense of urgency in persuading me to put Mom's Maryland home up for sale in May 2010, when Mom still seemed relatively healthy? The sale of her home was accomplished in November, the last month of her life when her health was touch-and-go. Diane also suggested I set up local bank accounts for Mom, which enabled my brother and me to distribute her cash assets in the end without a lawyer as she no longer had any tangible assets. Her house was sold and personal property shared according to her wishes. This avoided a lot of lawyer fees. Listen to that inner voice that prompts one to do things with sudden urgency.

Many other angel-like friends came alongside of us: Elaine, who looked in on Mom when she was at the Annapolis rehabilitation center '07 and took Mom's laundry home; Val, who took Mom to a Christmas party in Hawaii when I couldn't attend, and Catherine, who took Mom to a movie when her adult center was closed and

I had to teach. Sharon, our neighbor, played games and cards with Mom on occasion; and Ann, Catherine, and Bernie agreed to be on Mom's emergency list at the adult day care center. Kalei and her boys were so kind and ever entertaining to Mom, as she truly loved children. They, too, were a huge help in our last few months on the island. I found the most helpful people with Mom had gone through a similar experience themselves or couldn't be there to help their own parents at the time, and this was a wonderful way to help someone else.

I'll never forget that our neighbor Heidi in Colorado asked how she could help as Mom was dying, and I told her if she could bring her three young girls over to visit Mom, she would love that–and she did! Fred and Carol came over one evening so we could go to church together and the bonus was that our son Peter was visiting, and we were all able to attend church together. Another neighbor in Colorado, Margie, whom at that point we only saw while walking our dogs, also offered her help in those final days. The following week and the eve of her homegoing, Margie came so we could again regain some strength and refresh our souls in church. Remember to not neglect your body, mind, and spirit while on this difficult journey.

In 2011, after mom's death, Pete and Jess ran in the Denver Rock-N-Roll marathon to help raise funds for the Alzheimer's Association. It was Pete's first marathon since his motorcycle accident in Hawaii, a good test of his repaired leg, and Jess was running her first half marathon. At a point in the race when they were both tiring, a middle-aged man came from behind, running at a good clip and seemingly out of nowhere. Mom's name was printed on both their shirts as they were running in her memory. He shouted Mom's name over and over, cheering them on while passing them and suddenly disappearing into the crowd of runners. He came along at just the right time...angel?

Embrace the angels or perhaps just angelic friends God sends to you just when you need them most. They are all around you... and not always seen.

HELPFUL HINTS

Ask close friends who have met your loved one and have a connection with them to be on your emergency backup lists.

Consider putting a friend or two on legal/medical lists if you are the only living relative and or caretaker of your loved one.

Carry spare supplies in your car, i.e. wipes, a First Aid kit, adult diapers, towel and a change of clothes. Thankfully, my mom was usually continent, but the restaurant experience taught us, as my 'ole Girl Scout motto stated, to "be prepared."

Chapter 12
HOME CARE & OTHER OPTIONS

According to renowned journalist Andy Rooney, "A writer's job is to tell the truth," which he spoke on his <u>60 Minutes</u> episode entitled "Last Words." He died several weeks later.

So, this is my most important chapter because it will be quite simply, THE TRUTH. If you are giving care in your home to a loved one, as we did for my mom for two years while living in Hawaii, there may come a time for the sake of your mental, physical, and or emotional health that you need to find an alternative. Do not feel guilty.

If you remember nothing else from this book, remember this - NO ONE WILL CARE FOR YOUR LOVED ONE LIKE YOU WOULD. No one has the love or devotion or knows them as well as you do. Another caregiver doesn't know the history of their likes, dislikes, medical history, allergies, etc. Don't get me wrong - there are great caregivers out there who are willing to learn these things, who are darn near saintly, and I've met a couple of them. Sometimes I have wondered if those two weren't angels- literally. They are extremely rare because for many caregivers, I believe, it is just a "job."

So, when Dr. Mark told us that it was time to move Mom to "assisted living" during our move from Hawaii to Colorado in the summer of 2009, we heard him. He saw the disease progressing and what it was doing to us emotionally and physically after her living in our home for two years. He stated that when we went on our house hunting trip, we should also find a place for Mom. She was not to stay in the hotel with us or our new home. Change is extremely difficult for those with dementia, so when we landed in Colorado, the first stop, after the long night on the red eye, was to her new home.

God directed us to an old friend Diane who was living in Colorado and knew about dementia facilities from personal experience. So, on our one week house hunting trip in June '09 with the help of a great realtor, we found a dream home for us and an assisted living home for Mom. We also purchased furniture for Mom's place which was delivered, and had everything set up for her arrival in just a few weeks. However, Pete was not on board. He asked, "How can you do this?" I looked at him as though he had lost his mind. Maybe I was temporarily blinded, but I saw a beautiful facility that I thought would give her a bit more independence, which she wanted, and some activities as well. Pete didn't see it that way and dreaded the day we would leave her there.

Upon our return from the house hunting week, we did the best we could to prepare her for her new home. We took pictures of scenic Colorado, the house we purchased, and her new assisted living home. We showed her pictures of the beautiful garden area, porch, living room, dining room, and her new bedroom which was all set up. She seemed amenable to it, almost excited about the move. But I wasn't prepared for her reaction the day we left her there. Pete had anticipated it though.

There was another reason we were anxious to bring Mom to her assisted living center and not delay the move. Pete, in the exhaustion of preparing to move, doing his regular job as a Special Agent, and

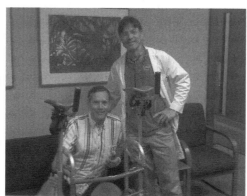

Pete with our doctor and his platform walker just before our move to Colorado

82

help with Mom, was utterly drained. This may have been a small part of the reason for his motorcycle accident. He arrived in Colorado sporting a platform walker due to broken ribs and collarbone, as well as, leg and hand surgery. Now Jess and I needed to concentrate on his recovery.

Our God-sent friend Diane and her son-in-law met us at the airport with two vehicles to help us transport our cat, dog, and 13 pieces of luggage which had to suffice the four of us for up to two months while waiting for the rest of our things to arrive

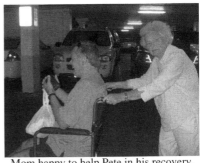
Mom happy to help Pete in his recovery.

from Hawaii. I told Mom to push Pete's wheelchair in the airport for a bit-if that wasn't a sight! She replied, "Why, sure!" and eagerly helped her son-in-law who was now in need of so much help himself. For the few minutes that she pushed him, Pete feared for his life, but she did the task with great pride. Jess and the pets went to the hotel, while Pete and I went with Mom. When we arrived at her new home, she followed me around like a duckling explaining how she didn't want to be left there: she didn't belong with "those" other people. It was absolutely heart-wrenching.

We were told not to come back until Mom had adjusted. I called daily to hear of her progress. One day we were told she attempted to escape by climbing the courtyard fence. Picture Mom throwing her purse down and attempting to scale a board-on-board fence! Also she wasn't interacting with others or eating well. On day ten, the activities director felt Mom was ready to see us. The activities director took the blame for us not visiting sooner, explaining we weren't "allowed." Mom was happy to see us, and we took her out to dinner. Our next concern was whether there would be a scene upon returning Mom to her new home. Instead, she just wanted to know when we would be back. Mom was adjusting to her new home. We were even allowed to bring her favorite dog Holly during our next visit!

Jess had come to Colorado only for the summer. She and Mom had a very close bond, but it was time for Jess to return to her life in Hawaii. It was a heart wrenching, "So long", as I was taught to say growing up. Goodbye is a forever phrase, "So long" meant "Until we meet again."

Now when I refer to "assisted living," I mean it gave the appearance of assisted living in every way, except when you tried to go out of any exit, alarms would sound. Fortunately, or unfortunately, Mom's new home had a plaque on the outside of the building which read, "Dementia and Memory Care" which we went to great lengths to prevent her seeing and reading.

We liked to take Mom out to dinner at least once a week, as dining out was one of her favorite things. Note - it is important to check for undergarments before leaving the nursing home! On one occasion, I noticed she did not have on her Depends as usual. It seemed as if she had found a pair of her underpants which we had gone to great lengths to hide. We took off Mom's pants to figure out the mystery. Well, to our surprise, she had put on one of her sleeveless undershirts. She had used the armholes for the legs, neckline for the waist, and as she stood up, the wadded-up body portion fell between her legs! Disaster averted!

On another occasion, checking for undergarments, we found she didn't have any on at all because she didn't "have any"...meaning she couldn't find her actual underpants and didn't realize there was a drawer full of Depends. But probably Pete's favorite undergarment check was when we discovered Mom wearing three Depends at one time! She was wearing one in traditional fashion, and two "sidesaddle" so to speak. We never did figure out how she was able to do that, as Pete had to literally cut the sideways ones off of her body!

One day, upon our return from another outing, it took some time for someone to come to the door and let us into the secure assisted living home. Mom spotted the sign and read it aloud questioningly. "Dementia and Memory Care?" she said in disbelief. Oh, boy, I had not anticipated this one, and I had to think fast. I said something like perhaps there were some people with memory problems who lived there. She gave me the look of disbelief and rolled her eyes. Then she muttered something about it "all making sense" with regard to some of the residents there. In a home with around 15 residents, there were only three of them including Mom, who were "with it" enough to pass off not being demented-until you spoke with them awhile. They were the most capable. This private assisted living home we chose was nicer than others we had ever seen or visited over many years with the Pets on Wheels Program.* It was a beautiful facility, with a maximum of 20 residents and was very cozy. In all appearances it was idyllic.

It only took a few weeks of visiting often to begin to see that the care was not what they said it would be. The staff had said Mom could attend some of the activities in another residential home, such as bridge and Bible study, but that never happened. In fact, there were no routine activities like Mom had in the center back in Hawaii. Upon our frequent visits we saw none of the promised purposeful brain exercises or activities, at least for the first several months. Then a new activities director came, and she was another "angel." Julianna planned activities, crafts, an occasional movie night with popcorn, and other social interactions. In talking with Julianna, a very spiritual person, I believe she felt part of her mission was to help make the transition from this life to the next for those in her loving care.

We brought Mom's many medications, 14 in all, to the nursing home monthly. We would give the new bottles, and a worker would give us the old bottles. This is when we noticed that not only were there leftovers of each medicine, but some had a lot left. For example, Namenda and Aricept were not being dosed properly, which was crucial. Once one is put on that medicine, it is essential to take it as prescribed and never go off it, for it helps slow down the disease. We had a meeting with the administrator regarding this and somehow walked away with the feeling that complaining would get us nowhere, except a new home elsewhere for Mom---the last thing she needed because she was beginning to make friends. Perhaps there were problems with Mom's meds because workers, with no nursing degree (LPN/RN) were handing out medications. Most of these workers had difficulty with the English language. Never assume nurses give medicine; ask questions.

Next we noticed laundry problems, which never should have happened, based on the fact that we were told by administrators that her laundry would be done separately. How on earth then was it that every time we visited, she had others' clothes in her closet? One time we noticed that Mom's salmon colored sweatshirt, a gift from my brother, was being worn by another resident! Oh, my! Pete had to literally hold me back from ripping it off the poor woman who had absolutely no clue it was my mother's sweatshirt. I can actually imagine my mom complimenting the other woman wearing the sweatshirt (not knowing it was hers), both of them in their own little world, as she loved that particular color.

Billing can be another area of concern. We questioned several thousand dollars of billing to Medicare for skilled nursing and therapeutic services. We did not understand why Mom needed these services, and ultimately Medicare did not pay the home for them. If you don't understand for what you are being billed, ask the facility financial director to explain in detail. If it doesn't make sense, call or write Medicare until you have an answer.

We would often visit around dinnertime and sit with Mom while she ate. It was then that we noticed that the staff had no understanding of ulcerative colitis or diabetes. I gave the staff a list of foods that triggered diarrhea, which you would think they would like to follow, considering the ensuing explosion they would have to clean up! Mom could not tolerate many milk products and spicy food. I really was never concerned about the small amounts of sugar in the desserts; after all, it was the little joy she had in life, and her sugar was generally controlled in the absence of infection. We know they gave her milk products, which we constantly had to re-explain to the foreign caregivers. On one such occasion, we watched them take away a small piece of cake and give her "sugar free" ICE CREAM! Ice cream was on the list of foods that would surely trigger an explosion... I felt so bad for Mom, because she was relatively continent when she kept to the foods she could eat. When Mom did have an accident, she was mortified, and it would often end up with her in unnecessary tears.

On one occasion while we were visiting Mom, she told us she needed to get back to her apartment to make dinner for Dad. I tried to gently explain that her meals were cooked for her there and that Dad had been dead for years. As usual, she looked to Pete as the only truth teller, and he nodded in agreement. She thought about it for several minutes and then said, "Then who was I sleeping with last night?" We suspected the new resident, who resembled my dad.

Showers were not given frequently enough as far as we were concerned, and we told the administration. I know they were concerned about frail skin and a dry climate, a particular problem in Colorado. We requested a brief shower every other day because of the chronic UTI's Mom had had since childhood. It seemed to be a physiological "plumbing problem", as Pete once encountered during a trip to Dr. Mark when Mom was still living with us. Mom no longer understood how to pee in a cup. Pete remarked on one occasion that he never had to hold a cup for me as he had to for Mom. He further remarked that Mom peed and sprayed like a fire sprinkler going off, and it was certainly difficult even for him to get it in the cup. I think I could have lived forever without that information, and I know Pete could have lived without that experience being seared in his memory!

A shower incident was the beginning of the end for Mom. Two male aides were helping Mom take a shower early one morning in mid-September 2010. The first problem was that Mom didn't want men helping her, and the second was that her body was in too much pain early in the morning. She tried to kick one of the aides, which caused a flesh tear to her weak skin. After the flesh tear she exhibited brief, stroke-like symptoms which landed her in the hospital for several days of testing and treating infection. At the end of her stay, it was agreed that her cardiologist would change her pacemaker battery in the hospital, as it was due to be changed anyway. Either in the operating room or during her stay at the rehabilitation nursing home, Mom contracted the deadly infection Methicillin-resistant Staphylococcus aureus (MRSA)** - which was the beginning of the end.

Mom had a generally happy experience at her assisted living place, despite the many problems she never realized were occurring. However, Mom did become fearful of one of the male employees which was why we were going to move her after her rehabilitation. She was scheduled to move to an even smaller, peaceful group home in the countryside recommended by her new doctor at the assisted living home. Mom would have a beautiful view on a golf course. I had also considered getting an apartment a few blocks away from our home and hiring our own employees to care for Mom there. My dear friend Gretchen had done this for her mom after having problems in a nursing home in another state. This was very successful for Gretchen and less costly than a nursing or group home. Find what will suit your loved one best.

 HELPFUL HINTS

*Pets on Wheels is a program for which we volunteered for many years while living in Maryland. Registered pets could visit nursing homes, which most of the residents loved. We visited on a weekly basis for many years.

**MRSA Methicillin-resistant Staphylococcus aureus is a more difficult staph to treat because it is resistant to commonly used antibiotics and is also known as the "super bug."

To find a good nursing home, visit several times before signing a contract. Ask questions about how often a nurse is on duty and whether they are the ones to distribute meds. Ask about male aides and if there is always a female on duty if your loved one has a preference. Ask about laundry procedures, how the staff is informed about food allergies, wandering, stealing, etc.

Consider a small group home but research it as well.

Review all bills especially the ones Medicare pays. Make sure the services were rendered and /or authorized by you.

Consider leasing an apartment close to your home and hiring your own staff. Perhaps you know someone who would like to have free room and board and a small paycheck to boot. This can usually be accomplished for less money than a group or nursing facility. Get the social security number of any employee you are considering and get a background check for peace of mind.

In some states, if you are caring for your loved one at home, you can be paid, which was brought to my attention after we had cared for Mom for over two years. Check with your states' nursing and licensure laws.

Chapter 13
END SIGNS

Mom's "best girlfriend" Jess moved home from Hawaii to live with us in Colorado in June of 2010. We had no idea what a God-send that was soon to be.

While visiting Mom in September 2010 at her assisted living home, one of our favorite employees engaged us in conversation. She noted that Mom had become less social and was sleeping more. A few months before she had been quite social when she had imagined that the three foot tall snowman we had bought her was a real child! She even fed him pretzels, which, when "he was full," we would find dangling from his nose. She would tell people that she could not attend activities because she had to "baby-sit the little boy in her room." It was suggested to us that Mom would probably die in her sleep one day before too long. During our nine day hospice experience, hospice personnel explained that in the dying process, sleep is the way one prepares to die. It is a way of reviewing one's life, thinking through the idea of dying, and preparing for the next life. The sleep factor and change in socializing were huge signs.

People with dementia typically also have a condition known as Sundowner's Syndrome.* Typically, when the sun goes down, your loved one may become significantly more confused or agitated. My mother did not suffer from this initially but began to more in the last year of her life and, in particular, during the last couple of months of her life. This confused nighttime behavior increased during her final months.

Another clue that your loved one is nearing the end of his/her life is that he/she will eat and drink less. Food loses its taste, and eating becomes a chore. This can be a very gradual process as it was in my mom's situation. You may even see confusion regarding the use of utensils and actually how to begin the process of eating!

God gave our family an incredible gift. In the last couple of months, particularly the last few weeks, we had several LUCID, dementia free conversations. I am told that these types of clear conversations in dementia patients are not unusual near the end of life, so what a gift! It's almost as if Mom knew she was dying and mustered a few moments of common sense for a short period of time in order to share a message regarding her death.

Just about two months before she died, Mom told Jessica that she was dying. She wanted her to know that she was dying and not to be upset about it. She didn't want Jess to alarm others by telling us either. She proceeded to tell her that it was OK and that she was not afraid to die. This was the first time she had peace about the process. She asked Jess, "Will people miss me?" and "Will I be remembered?" She asked those two questions several times in the last few months of her life. We reassured her that, indeed, she would be missed and, of course, she would be remembered. If you had ever known my mom, you would know it would be impossible to forget her. It was a precious conversation that they shared that night. Jess called me from the nursing home that night sobbing. Once I understand what she was saying, I urged her to write notes about the conversation they had. How I wished Pete was home, but he was away on a business trip. I asked her if she thought I should come right over, and after some thought we decided that Mom would probably not die that night. Jessica alerted the night nurse to keep an extra eye on Mom and to call us if there was any change. Mom was aware that she was, indeed, beginning the process of dying.

Mom had a rough time during the last couple of months of her life, beginning in September. A couple of days after a flesh tear of the leg, she had what appeared to be a mild stroke and another urinary tract infection (UTI).** This landed her in the hospital for a week. At the end of the week, she had a routine pacemaker battery change. Just as she came out of surgery and was being wheeled back to her room, I witnessed Mom trying to get a date with the male nurse wheeling her! Next, Mom went to regain her strength at a residential rehabilitation center. That stay turned into two months due to recurring UTI's and MRSA. The poor thing had been complaining regularly about the pacemaker wound which appeared to be healing nicely. However, unbeknownst to us, the antibiotics she was receiving for the UTI's had been keeping a growing infection in the new pacemaker, at bay. Suddenly, two months after the pacemaker surgery, it had swollen to the size of half a baseball sitting on her chest! Then the entire pacemaker had to be removed and replaced to treat the MRSA. However, the pacemaker had been in her for eight years, so it could not be easily removed! We had to find one of only a few doctors in the entire state of Colorado who could do the laser surgery to get the leads out. Just before the surgery, Mom told the x-ray tech who had to move and position her, which was uncomfortable, "It's time to go home. Your mother is calling you!" He got a chuckle out of that. We met nurse Michael just after the surgery, and Mom was reminiscing with him about the area they both came from in New York. He was a quick study of Mom, which is just one thing that made him an exceptional nurse. He began calling her "Gerdie," which was one of many nicknames we had for Mom. Our favorite old family names for Mom were "Gerdie" and "Sadie." She answered to all of them! After the new pacemaker was put in, the doctors inadvertently collapsed a lung. It was all too much for the old girl.

Since September we visited the hospital, rehabilitation center, and the second hospital (which was tasked with removing the previous pacemaker and wires) daily. I was there for lunch: Pete and Jessica tag-teamed for dinner time so we could encourage Mom to eat. Mom began to talk to the three of us about dying one day around Thanksgiving. We were so slap happy from sheer exhaustion that we didn't try to talk her out of it. So I pulled out my pocket calendar, and Jess turned to December 2010. I elbowed her arm and told her to switch it to November, but she didn't. Mom carefully reviewed the calendar and pointed December 26. Jess said, "December 26, right?" Mom nodded and smiled. So I replied, "Oh, you just want to get presents!" and she agreed. She still had a childlike joy in the celebration of Christmas.

It was nearly three weeks of Mom not gaining her strength back, when I had my "Ah ha moment." Dr. Christy came in and spoke with me. She began by apologizing that she was not good at "these types of conversations," so I knew I was not in for good news. She said she would like to be wrong concerning my mom but it was her belief that Mom was not going to get better. Yes, they had healed all infection, and the lung had almost completely re-inflated, but Mom was still dying. Failure to thrive is what it is commonly called. She then said the most meaningful thing any doctor had ever said concerning my mom. We could continue to treat her with IV fluids, tube feeding, etc. However, in doing so, "As doctors, we sometimes get in the way of God's plan for a peaceful exit," particularly when continually treating the elderly. Wow! My dilemma, as a Christian, had been to treat as long as treatment was available, yet she was saying that could be so much harder on Mom. For example, if Mom got aspiration pneumonia, that was a painful "exit." Nurse Michael paid her several visits even though he was not Mom's nurse anymore. He came from a Catholic background but simply agreed with Dr. Christy. He said, "Gerdie wouldn't want this", referring to any attempt to extend her life. In that short time he had read Mom well. After speaking with my pastor on several occasions and my brother, we agreed to bring Mom to our home with the help of hospice.***

I suddenly really saw that she was dying---it was truly as if blinders had been taken off my eyes! Mom almost made her goal of one last Christmas...

HELPFUL HINTS

*Sundowner's Syndrome-characterized by increased memory loss, confusion, and/or agitation in patients with dementia at sundown.

**UTI- urinary tract infection-commonly seen in those with suppressed immune systems. It has many causes but is more common in the elderly, particularly those in nursing homes. Dehydration and a genetic predisposition (shorter urethra) are factors. It increases confusion, especially in the elderly with or without dementia!

***Hospice specializes in both medical care and pain management. The focus is on comfort and death with dignity. Hospice's team-oriented approach of professionals supports the patient as well as the family.

The most important thing my nurse friend Ann told me was that when your loved one nears death's doorstep, it is important to reassure them that you will be OK when they die. Give them your permission to let go, to die!

Chapter 14
FINAL DAYS

Dr. Christy took the time to lovingly tell me that, in her professional opinion, there was nothing more they could do for Mom as doctors except to interfere with what would otherwise be a "peaceful exit."

During our teleconference, which included Pete, Jessica, my pastor, the palliative doctor, my brother, and me, I begged my older brother, Steve, to make the right decision concerning Mom's care and Living Will* wishes, as I still struggled with letting her go. It seemed to be a moral dilemma I could not get around, but intellectually I knew no further heroic action was what Mom wanted. We needed to let her go on

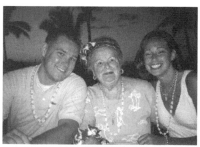

Our son Peter, Mom, and Jessica during healthier days.

her own terms. For example, I knew she needed IV fluids, but as the doctor and her favorite nurse Michael explained, it would most likely not change the outcome of what was happening. As her medical and financial representative, I also knew Mom did not want any life extending measures, such as CPR or tube feeding. So, what good would fluids actually do? Still, the moral dilemma for me was whether to stop treatment. Now, mind you, the MRSA was under control; she had finished antibiotics, the lung was almost completely re-inflated, but she still was not thriving. Thankfully, my brother Steve said the words we all needed to hear. "If my sister and her family are willing to take her [Mom] home in the care of hospice, then let's do that." I felt somewhat "off the hook" for the decision which is what we all agreed was the right thing to do.

Suddenly, I felt a sense of urgency regarding getting her to our home and preparing for her home-going--- to her Heavenly Father. We had the teleconference on Thursday, December 9, and, with the help of Mom's geriatrician, had hospice care and Mom in our home the next day.

I had hospice set Mom's hospital type bed up in the family room near the T.V. and in front of the fireplace which was next to a window. Our kitchen flowed into the family room which was the hub of our activity. It was the perfect place for Mom. She could look out the family room window and see people outside as there was a park and walking paths behind our house. She spoke about wanting to see snow, and God was gracious to grant that wish. Mom had childlike memories of making snow angels and recalled how the snow "went crunch, crunch" underfoot. Funny, I only remember her dislike for the messiness of snow and how she disliked driving in it!

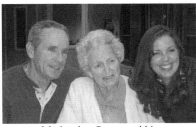
My brother Steve, and his daughter, Keri visit Mom

I called our son Peter Thursday night and told him it was time to come and see "Nanny" one more time. I explained with "now or never" urgency which I had never done before. He got a plane ticket and arrived Friday at the exact time we were arriving home with Mom from the hospital. I told my brother Steve, who had recently seen her, that if he wished to see her one last time---it was now! He arrived a couple of days after Peter's visit which gave her time in between visits to rest. Oh, how Mom rallied for those two visits by eating the best she could and trying to hold conversations with them both. It was a heaven-sent time for all.

We learned a lot in those nine short days about the death process and other practical things with the help of the hospice minister, nurses, and aides. One thing our hospice nurse explained was that during the times Mom was sleeping and unable to communicate, she could, indeed, hear us. Hospice also explained that dying patients could time their last breath to either have others around or spare them. They had seen families literally take turns sitting vigil over their loved one. Then, when the person sitting vigil got up briefly to go to the bathroom, the loved one would take his/her last breath. Conversely, sometimes the dying person would hold on for the last relative to arrive and have everyone around them. I was certain that Mom would die during the night as we all slept.

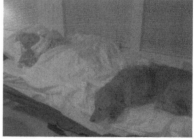
Holly welcoming Mom to our home

Nate, the pastor with hospice, came out to see Mom. They had a lovely, and again, lucid conversation. They spoke of her childhood and the fact that her dad, my grandfather, would sometimes preach in their hometown Methodist church. She recalled things in amazing detail. But what Mom wanted to talk about was her unfounded concern that, "She didn't know God." Raised in the church, I found this comment interesting. He proceeded to ask, "If Jesus were sitting here, what would you tell him?" She replied, "I love you." What an example of the childlike faith in which we enter the kingdom of heaven! (Matthew 18) I had been in the room or nearby as they spoke. Then Mom called me over and whispered loudly, "See that nice man? I don't want him to leave!" I reassured her that he was not leaving just yet, and she smiled and winked at him...FLIRT! He read her favorite passage from the Bible, Psalm 23, and she recited the words with him from memory.

Mad Cow Disease (Creutzfeldt-Jakob disease) is a
central nervous system disease affecting cows. Humans
can contract this disease by eating beef from an infected
cow. Cows are thought to contract this disease by eating
feed that has been contaminated with dead cows.

Hospice also made sure that we had our paperwork in
order, in particular, the proper HIPAA document in
which I was empowered to make medical decisions. We
also needed a copy of the Emergency Medical Services/
Do Not Resuscitate Medical Care Order in our home
in case one of us panicked and called an ambulance. It
had been my mother's wish not to be resuscitated, to
have an airway or tube feeding. But it was my mother's
wish to be an organ donor. Through hospice we learned
that people with dementia can NOT be organ donors!
This is because the symptoms of dementia mimic Mad
Cow Disease.** Interestingly enough, she spent several
months in England, eating beef in restaurants during the
Mad Cow outbreak! The only definitive way to diagnose
Alzheimer's disease or Mad Cow disease is to dissect the
brain. How disappointing it was that she could not help
others by donating usable body parts. It had been her
final wish.

So, in those final days, sometimes Mom would ask, "Am
I dying?" and other days she would tell us, "I am dying."
On December 16, she said, "God help me," as she quite
often did. This time we asked, "Help you with what?"
She replied, "God will help me to do whatever I need to
do." As I left for a hair appointment that same day, I
asked her if I had been a good daughter. She replied,
"Oh, sure, don't you worry about that," as the tears rolled
down my face. Seeing me getting sentimental, she said,
"Don't you cry, or I won't come back!" She was mothering
me for one final time.

Then on December 18, in another lucid moment she said,
"I love you so much. I love you so much I am scared that
something is 'gonna go bang'." I think she meant within
her body. And then she later told me that my deceased
father had called and "left a message."

On December 19, the day she died, she once again told Pete, "You're a good man, Pete Sackrider" and that was quite simply the truth. They had become very close over the three years. Pete had turned his love for Mom from family obligation to unconditional love and compassion for Mom. It was a beautiful sight. She was sleeping more that day but could still answer questions coherently. I had been thinking about her obituary for months but had ironically decided to start typing her obituary that day of all days! We were trying to figure out what year she had graduated high school and asked her, "1946 or 1947?" and she replied while almost completely asleep, "1946."

I found myself almost avoiding spending time with her because I knew something was different. When I did go over to speak with her to find out whether she needed anything to eat or drink, she replied, "Yes" but didn't take more than a sip. What she did do was rub my arm and hold my hand! In fact, it was a "death grip"! My fingers were red and throbbing from being held so tightly! I put my head gently on her chest and quietly sobbed during those final moments that she comforted me as she was slipping away.

Later that same afternoon, Mom said, "Something is happening, and I can't stop it," again referring to the dying process. That evening Pete had a sweet, very quiet conversation with Mom regarding his unconditional love and forgiveness toward her which she seemed to understand and appreciate. I know she must have heard us discussing that Pete had to go into work for a couple of hours. Around 8:00 pm shortly after Pete's private conversation, I reminded Pete that if he had work to do that he should get going and get back! So, around 8:30 he got his coat on and prepared to leave. I asked him to give Mom her pain meds before leaving and things suddenly and quickly began to change, so he did not leave.

His procrastination had paid off! Her breathing ha become labored, but she appeared to be in no pain. asked Pete to call hospice to see if there was anyth else we could give her for the labored breathing. I my arms around her from behind the bed and held o hand as Jess held the other, and Pete was standing her side on the phone with hospice. I wiped one sm tear from her eye. Mom was the type that hated t "miss anything," so in that respect it was still hard her to leave. To this day, Jessica and Pete think hi sweet little conversation with Mom triggered the fi events, somehow giving her the final permission to "

She no longer had the strength to grasp our hands as she had previously that day: they had gone limp. I grasped her hand and held on tightly to her as I f her begin to slip away. We very briefly prayed the p she taught me as a young child. "Now I lay me down sleep, I pray the Lord my soul to keep, If I should d before I wake, I pray the Lord my soul to take." We sang one of her favorite hymns, kissed her, and told we loved her one last time in those final moments as drifted into the arms of her Heavenly Father at 9:1 choosing family to surround her. It was peaceful, ar wasn't afraid. It was finished: her purpose here on e was now complete.

 HELPFUL HINTS

*Living Will is a legal document that a person uses to make known his/her wishes known regarding life prolonging medical treatments. It can be also known as an Advanced Directive, Health Care Directive, or Physician's Directive. It specifies what treatment yo do or do not want only when you become incapacitated make such decisions.

AFTERWORD

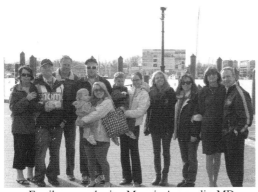

Family remembering Mom in Annapolis, MD

Three months after Mom's death, we took a cruise which was according to her wishes. She wanted her death to be a celebration of her life. She said, "Have a party!" Additionally, my brother saw to it that we followed the outline she had made for her own memorial service and party-which she had written in 2002! It was held at her home church in Annapolis and was a lovely celebration.

Ultimately, I have no regrets, but I do wish I had had the patience that Pete had with Mom. About a year after we had Mom in our home and her mental status was slowly declining, I realized that as an educator I was failing. I had never failed before. It caused some of my impatience with her, and although I understood intellectually, it didn't help. Many of these funny stories were not funny to Jessica and me at the time! We would explain to Pete that Mom was our shared bloodline. So the embarrassing moments and fear of a heredity/ lifestyle link with dementia was a concern to us. I am confident we did the absolute best we could, one day at a time, and learned about this disease as we went along. We learned through observation, doctors, and books.

It is difficult when you care for someone for over three years to suddenly stop. As the undertakers were wheeling Mom out of our home, I almost stopped them because it was 11:00pm---time for a bandage change.

Wow! That was a weird thought. And, three months after mom's death, Pete saw an empty pill container which we used to set up Mom's meds for the week. For a brief moment as he turned pale he thought, "Oh, no! I need to get her pills set up!"

Thankfully, hospice was there to help us through the grieving process---one you may not even know you are going through. After all, it was a relief after everything we had been through, right? But it was not so easy. We had lost a loved one. The stages of grieving are very similar, but there is no "normal" as to how people progress through them. If you suspect that someone is having difficulty with a loss, consult a professional. A dear friend told me, "We grieve so deeply because we loved so deeply."

Hospice talks about finding a "new normal" in one's life to fill the void. When we had moved to Colorado in 2009, I applied for part-time teaching positions so I could still be available to Mom. I was fortunate to find a tutoring position but with the slowing economy my hours dwindled. So, three months after Mom died, I found my "new normal," and after more than 25 years in education, I am beginning a new career in banking. And I thank Jesse, Josh, and Chelsea for thinking they could teach this "old dog new tricks."

I was able to get together with my dear friend Gretchen one evening while visiting our son and his family in Massachusetts in January, a month after Mom's death. Pete and I met Gretchen for dinner. She had cared for her mom with dementia for several years as well. We had many shared experiences. What was interesting was that she was absolutely exhausted for months after her mother's death. She said she took naps every day. Her body needed it. Hospice believes that the grief process is very individual and that people who even share the same loss progress through it differently. Listen to your heart and take care of your body through sleep and proper nutrition. My Aunt Barbara would tell you that tears made of salt water hold healing power!

Life is good.

Jessica and Mom had gone to see <u>The Bucket List</u> movie when it came out in 2007. That was probably the last movie that she comprehended. When she came home, she

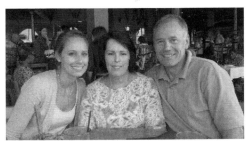
Jessica, me, and Pete, August 2013

said, "No one over the age of 70 should be allowed to see that movie. I don't know when I laughed so hard or cried so hard." Then I asked her if she had anything left on her bucket list. She replied something to this effect, "No, I've had a very good life. I've traveled and seen the world, had a good marriage, and raised two children. I've seen my grandchildren and great grandchildren. There is nothing left that I want to do." I thought to myself that this was, indeed, a good sign. Then a few days later she said, "I would like to see Jessica get married." But alas, there was not a suitor in sight!

During one of those last conversations I had with Mom as she was losing her "fight," I asked, "Don't you want to live to see Jessica get married?" She simply replied, "Tell her I am tired of waiting." Oh, there were a number of occasions during those years that we thought... if we could just complete the bucket list, maybe she would feel that she could die. So we would scheme about how we could hire actors or perhaps ask a boyfriend to pretend to marry Jessica. But we just couldn't do it! Now, I look at future suitors through a different lens. I wonder to myself, "Will you help to care for me when I no longer can? Help me shower? Hold my hand? Be patient with me?" I believe there were only a few times that Pete got stern with Mom. They were the times Mom thought she was married to him. Pete would firmly reply in a booming voice, "WE WERE NEVER MARRIED!" As Pete often said, "I never signed up for this when we got married." Yet, he had the patience of Job.

Colton Burpo recounted in his story "Heaven Is for Real" that during his brief visit to heaven, he met Jesus first and that everyone in heaven had a "job." I envision Mom as having a playgroup of children around her as she loved children! And every time I hear Bart Miller's song, "I Can Only Imagine," I think of Mom flashing a wide smile with her deep dimples upon meeting Jesus and giving that "nice man" a huge wink!

A few days after Mom died and I was sobbing, it came to me. It was as though I had suffered not only the loss of my mother but it felt like the death of a child !

We had come full circle, and now the circle was complete.

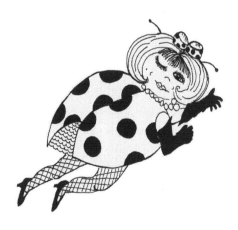

Footprints in the Sand

One night I dreamed I was walking along the beach with the Lord.
Many scenes from my life flashed across the sky.
In each scene I noticed footprints in the sand.
Sometimes there were two sets of footprints, other times there were one set of footprints.

This bothered me because I noticed
that during the low periods of my life,
when I was suffering from
anguish, sorrow or defeat,
I could see only one set of footprints.

So I said to the Lord,
""You promised me Lord,
that if I followed you,
you would walk with me always.
But I have noticed that during the most trying periods of my life
there have only been one set of footprints in the sand.
Why, when I needed you most, you have not been there for me?""

The Lord replied,
""The times when you have seen only one set of footprints, is when I carried you.""

© *Mary Stevenson*

SUGGESTED READING

The 36 Hour Day Nancy L. Mace M.A. and Peter V. Rabbins, MD., M.P.H.

The Forgetting Alzheimer's Portrait of an Epidemic by David Shenk

Losing My Mind by Thomas DeBaggio

Twilight Travels with Mother by Mary Ann Mayo

Alzheimer's Early Stages by Daniel Khun, MSW

Mayo Clinic Guide to Alzheimer's Disease

APPENDIX

LEGAL TERMS:

Advanced Health Care Directive - also known as a Living Will. This document is to be used in the event that your loved one can no longer make decisions for his/herself. It names an "agent" to make specific health care decisions on their behalf.

EMS and DNR Order - This is a free document you can get from your loved one's doctor which states their medical wishes for EMS-Emergency Medical Services concerning DNR-Do Not Resuscitate. This website from Maryland explains more fully www.miemss.umaryland.edu/ (The three states in which we cared for Mom, (MD, HI, and CO) required this separate document. It allows the ambulance crew to follow your loved one's wishes. POA and HIPAA documents do not cover the ambulance trip.)

Family and Medical Leave Act of 1993 - (signed by President Clinton) provides up to 12 weeks of unpaid, job-protected leave per year while caring for a family member and other personal or family related medical situations.

Health Insurance Portability and Accountability Act of 1996 - **(HIPAA)** This act was established for the privacy of individually identifiable health information and for proper use of the sharing of protected health information among health professionals. (It is important to legally document specific people who can have access to and make decisions concerning your loved one's health.)

Living Trust - A legal document that protects your loved one's assets for his/her use while they are living, then any remaining assets are transferred to their beneficiaries upon his/her death.

Living Will - a legal document that a person uses to make known his/her wishes known regarding life prolonging medical treatments. It can be also known as an Advanced Directive, Health Care Directive, or Physician's Directive. It specifies what treatment you do or do not want only when you become incapacitated to make such decisions.

Power of Attorney - a legal document authorizing one to represent or act on another's behalf in private, business or other legal matters. (This document enabled me to sell my mother's home when it became apparent that she could no longer live on her own.)

Will - a legal document drafted and executed according to state law and is irrevocable upon death. It states how your loved one wishes their assets to be divided. (I suggest you consult a lawyer specializing in estate planning for guidance on this.)

MEDICAL TERMS:

Alzheimer's Disease - Accounting for up to 80% of all dementia cases, it is the most common form of dementia and worsens over time. It is associated with plaques and tangles in the brain. It is the sixth leading cause of death in the US.

Cellulitis - a bacterial infection, usually strep or staph, obtained through an opening in the skin such as a cut or even an insect bite which spreads to deeper tissues. People with weak immune systems, diabetes, and peripheral arterial disease are particularly susceptible. The infected area can be warm, red, and tender. Fever and chills may follow. Left untreated, it can lead to death.

Dementia - Dementia is the general term for loss of

cognitive brain function due to damaged brain cells which occur with certain diseases and is not a part of normal ageing process. Dementia affects memory, language, judgment, thinking and behavior. It interferes with daily living.

Frontotemporal Dementia - Also known as Pick's disease and is similar to Alzheimer's disease except that is only affects the frontal and temporal lobes of the brain. This disease worsens slowly.

Lewy Body Dementia - This form of dementia is closely associated with dementia and Parkinson's disease. Cognition and alertness fluctuate daily or hourly with possible hallucinations. They can think people or animals are present when they are not. Problems with vision may occur misinterpreting what they see. Unusual gait, stiff movements, blank stare, difficulty swallowing may be present.

Mad Cow Disease (Creutzfeldt-Jakob disease) - Is a central nervous system disease affecting cows. Humans can contract this disease by eating beef from an infected cow. Cows are thought to contract this disease by eating feed that has been contaminated with dead cows.

MRSA - Methicillin-resistant Staphylococcus aureus - A more difficult staph to treat because it is resistant to commonly used antibiotics and is also known as the "super bug."

MMSE - Mini-Mental State Examination an excellent barometer of whether one may be in early stages of dementia can be found online. Copyright: M. Folstein, S Folstein, P MCHugh. See example: enotes.tripod.com/MMSE.pdf

PAD - Peripheral Artery Disease - Mayo Clinic describes as a circulatory problem in which narrowed arteries reduce the blood flow to limbs. It often may be a sign to more widespread fatty deposits (plaques) in arteries which can lead to atherosclerosis. This can cause reduced blood flow to the brain.

POCD - Postoperative Cognitive Dysfunction - a temporary cognitive decline (brain fog) due to the effects of anesthesia which may be a more permanent cognitive loss in the elderly or those with dementia.

Sundowner's Syndrome - characterized by increased memory loss, confusion, and/or agitation in patients with dementia at sundown.

TIA's - Transient Ischemic Attacks - also known as 'mini strokes'

tPA - Tissue Plasminogen Activator - a drug which must be administered within a few hours after documenting a stroke or heart attack has occurred. It breaks up the clot which caused the event. The use of tPA can be fatal.

UTI - Urinary Tract Infection - an infection commonly seen in those with suppressed immune systems. It has many causes but is more common in the elderly, particularly those in nursing homes. Dehydration and a genetic predisposition (shorter urethra) are factors. It increases confusion, especially in the elderly with or without dementia.

Vascular Dementia - Occurs when blood vessels are damaged and reduce circulation to the brain, vital oxygen and nutrients are deprived from the brain as well. Vascular dementia can also occur after a stroke blocks an artery to the brain. Risk factors include high blood pressure, high

7850584R00064

Made in the USA
San Bernardino, CA
19 January 2014

cholesterol, untreated thyroid problems, and smoking.

LESS COMMON CAUSES OF DEMENTIA:
*Traumatic brain injury
*Parkinson's disease
*Huntington's disease
*Creutsfeldt-Jakob disease also known as Mad Cow
  disease
*Acquired Immunodeficiency Syndrome-AIDS

POTENTIALLY REVERSABLE CAUSES OF DEMENTIA:
(consult your doctor)

*Depression
*Adverse effects of drugs
*Normal Pressure Hydrocephalus (NPH)
*Vitamin deficiencies, such as B12
*Severe Thyroid disease
*Excess alcohol